"Dwayne J. Clark has long been a pioneer in the fields of health and longevity. His hard-won wisdom speaks to all of us, irrespective of age. 30 Summers More is more than a key to the healthy-living treasure chest: it is a key to a chest full of health-promoting keys. Your journey to optimum health begins here".

Dr. Kirtland C. Peterson
Author of Post-Traumatic Stress Disorder: A Clinician's Guide

"When there is so much darkness in the world Dwayne Clark is a shining light with his undying efforts to change the world through compassion and empathy. A true example of the American dream."

Michael Bennett
Football Defensive End for the New England Patriots

"Dwayne's passion for you to live a healthier, happier, more fulfilling life comes through in every page of this book. As a student of health and longevity, I love the 30 Summers More formula for a life full of purpose, curiosity and enduring health."

Wes Moss
Financial Advisor, Author and host of Money Matters

"Dwayne breaks down the complex process of healthy living for longevity into actionable bite-sized nuggets of delicious truths. Even if you only apply 20% of the actionable items you will experience and feel the benefits in your day to day life."

Dr. Steve Young
Serial Entrepreneur with three decades of innovation in longevity and healing

"Dwayne Clark's globetrotting exploration into the universal and timeless qualities of aging well allows the reader to develop their personal owner's manual for late-life growth and happiness. However, this wise book isn't just for those at the end of their lifespan. His approach to the creation of a physically healthy, mentally resilient, and purpose driven way of living can be put into action at any point, from our youth onward."

Dr. Glen Hammel
Geriatric Neuropsychologist and Well-Aging Specialist

"Our culture is in desperate need of leadership that can promote the changes that Dwayne inculcates. Dwayne is very relatable and is breaking through barriers with lifestyle change that the next generation can follow! Don't put off tomorrow what you can do today and pickup a copy of Dwayne's book, "30 Summers More".

Gwen Rich
Founder of The Rich Solution and Wall Street Journal best-selling author of
Stop Complaining Make Your Own Luck

30 SUMMERS MORE

ADDING TIME BACK TO YOUR AGING CLOCK

Dwayne J. Clark

FILMMAKER, AUTHOR, PLAYWRIGHT, AND PHILANTHROPIST

Dwayne J. Clark

FILMMAKER, AUTHOR, PLAYWRIGHT, AND PHILANTHROPIST

Also by Dwayne J. Clark:

Help Wanted: Recruiting, Hiring
& Retaining Exceptional Staff

My Mother, My Son

Saturdays With GG

A Big Life: Wisdom for My Grandchildren

Printed in the United States of America

First printing, 2019

978-1-944194-62-8

Aegis Living
415 118th Ave SE
Bellevue, WA 98005

MEDICAL DISCLAIMER

The material presented in this book is for informational purposes only and is not intended to serve as a substitute for the consultation, diagnosis, or medical treatment of a qualified physician or health care provider.

Contents

*All profits from the primary sale of this book
will be donated to charity.*

To Frank Burke

1953-2018

To a good friend, father, writer, and
a man's man who left us far too soon.

Foreword

Dr. Ordon

As I continue my journey in life, I am confident that there is still a lot of life to live. So much left to see and experience! My ability to live longer is greater than I ever imagined possible. I've led a fantastic life and plan on doubling down in my next thirty summers on this planet!

Longevity is truly a passion of mine and one of the core pillars of my life's work. As a doctor, better health through medical advancements is hardcoded into our DNA. As a husband and father of two, life is about maximizing the quality of time spent with those most important to me. Through knowledge and action, the defenders of longevity, I have been able to maximize my future experiences while minimizing the struggles we all face as we age. In the grandest way, life is not as much about where you are going, but more about the journey; it can be long and exciting or cut short due to pain. The choice is ours.

Having finished medical school over 30 years ago, I have come to appreciate the day-to-day experiences which define our purpose which changes as we age. Education isn't over when you get your diploma. I've never stopped learning or evolving my knowledge and practices. Even preparing for my daily appearances on "The Doctors" is like preparing for exams in medical school. Always learning. This constant desire for self improvement is one that lasts for a lifetime as a physician.

Sharing my knowledge to impact the lives of others is something I've been blessed to do in my medical practice, my work on television, and in my charitable work. My view of what it means to be a doctor has changed over the years. I once believed my job was to 'fix and heal' people physically. Now, I see my role to teach others how to take charge of their health – to take charge both physically and emotionally – a balance that allows the inside to support the outside. Healthcare should not be synonymous with triage but with vibrancy.

Being on the Emmy-winning television show "The Doctors over the past decade has opened many doors for me personally and professionally. One of the biggest is my opportunity to travel the world as a volunteer with charitable organizations; sharing my knowledge and lending my skills. I went to India with Smile Train in 2010 performing cleft lip and palate procedures for a population that is in dire need of these services. I've traveled the world in this capacity ever since. This is where my professional expertise and my passionate purpose come together perfectly. Strengthening my soul by helping others.

Meeting Dwayne J. Clark was another door opened. Not a doctor himself, instead he is a longevity explorer, we are teachers with a shared mission. Let me rewind the clock a bit on how our stories intertwine.

About the same time, I began in medicine, Dwayne started his work in the assisted living industry. While caring for patients in surgery, hospital beds, in private practice, on television and in my missionary work, Dwayne was taking care of his senior residents in different ways. As the Founder of Aegis Living, Dwayne has set a culture of education with his staff making them more committed to helping their residents. His one-of-a-kind facilities resemble luxury anti-aging resorts with a focus on anti-aging practices and social interaction; both proven to extend life.

Like me, Dwayne travels extensively in search of knowledge that can help us live better - body, mind, spirit. Funny, that we get connected at this stage in our lives where we value our similar purpose above all.

Dwayne and I share a deeply personal connection to our mother's. Dwayne and I are unknowingly brothers of the same fraternity - the one for sons who have had to watch their mother pass too early. My mother, stricken with Dementia, while Dwayne's mother was overcome by Alzheimer's, we watched, helpless. When you witness a parent you've loved deeply and respected your entire life become a shadow of their once vibrant self; it changes you. Your direction, focus, and purpose on the planet are forever altered.

As the Founder of Aegis Living, Dwayne stands at the front line of the aging community, witnessing such terrible diseases such as Dementia and Alzheimer's wreak havoc on the lives of his residents. The pain of watching some go through it is indescribable. Research in the field of preventing Dementia and Alzheimer's is one that I especially champion and having Dwayne in the fight is critical.

30 Summers More is a fantastic compilation of how to seek out and cherish longevity – imagine watching the sun rise and set for years longer than you believe – filled with purpose and joy. This book is deeply personal, refreshingly presented, and extensively researched. His point of view on longevity is a call-to-action for all of us. He does not pretend to offer medical advice or beg for you to follow a specific diet and lifestyle. 30 Summers aligns purpose with health to provide lifestyle possibilities. Like I often do on "The Doctors," Dwayne uses personal stories to

educate and details the health experiments he has performed on himself – it's packed with "longevity hacks." He urges you not to 'give into midlife'; warns not to overwork yourself into death. He passionately conveys that no one has a life sentence to their current state of health happiness. He pulls together chapters filed with research and case studies that clearly show that aging and illness do not have to go hand-in-hand. Readers are encouraged to make a deep connection with their doctors; rather than pulling people into a set philosophy of alternative health only. True to his life as an educator and mentor, he coaxes the reader into becoming a life-long learner and to never stop applying new lessons in our lives.

This book delivers a powerful combination of how 40, 50, 60, 70, 80-year-olds can achieve a healthy edge while being inspired by their own life's purpose. He encourages us to create 'living artifacts' with our creative endeavors, our philanthrophy, our care for one another, and our constant investment in ourselves – proof that we are enjoying our time on this planet and leaving moments, experiences, and pathways for those who will come after us!

The underlying theme is to live a long and meaningful life. Before agreeing to perform any plastic surgery on a patient, I always ask them 'why.' Why are they altering their "outside." First and foremost, people have to be coming to be for the right reasons; perhaps bringing back some confidence they might have been lost. Our outside can be perfect, but if our inside (body, soul, and mind) are unhealthy, we will never be truly happy. It doesn't make a difference how handsome, pretty, or how young you look if you don't live a long and meaningful life. On top of taking care of your general health, as Dwayne has discovered, having a purpose in life is imperative to longevity. Bravo!

Imagine if my mother, Dwayne's mother, maybe your mother had access to this type of information BEFORE illness became stronger than life...

Dwayne and I both share this mission; life should be long and spectacular. Learn, act, live!

You'll be doing yourself and your family a huge favor by absorbing and practicing what you uncover in this book. Implement a single idea from Dwayne's journey, and you'll be on the road to living in the NOW, living WELL, and living LONGER.

In good health,

Andrew P. Ordon, M.D.,F.A.C.S.
Board Certified Plastic Surgeon, and
Associate Professor of Plastic Surgery, Keck/USC School of Medicine
Host, The Doctors TV

Acknowledgments

All books are a journey. This one has been five years in the making. It has involved travel to observe and meet people from around the world; hours of reading, studying, and interviewing; personal experiments with pills, supplements, diets, and all kinds of traditional and holistic practices; and the time and commitment of all the people I asked, cajoled, questioned, and enlisted to share their knowledge, skill, curiosity, and critical thinking in the development of the ideas and the writing of this book.

Early in the project, I enlisted the collaboration of Shirley Newell, MD, who is my colleague, and Aegis Living's chief medical officer. She's a triple-board-certified physician and has been a gerontologist for many decades. I'm indebted to her for the role she took in managing the research, making sense of the latest thinking and studies on healthy aging, and helping shape the themes and habits that became the heart of the book. She traveled to conferences, interviewed leading experts, and was an invaluable sounding board and thinking partner as I connected my personal story, professional experiences, and a lifetime of acquired knowledge with the newest discoveries about the intersection of our habits and our health. Shirley was absolutely indispensable in the creation of this book.

Partway into the project, Shirley brought Julie Hunt, PhD, on board as a health researcher to make sure we had the highest caliber information. Julie worked on the Women's Health Initiative at the Fred Hutchinson Cancer Research Center for many years and brought experience designing and analyzing research. She was instrumental in tracking down and making sense of the evolving science that was proving the impact of our lifestyles and environments on our health.

Judy Meleliat is my friend and president of Aegis. She was a fantastic facilitator in getting *30 Summers More* to completion. Judy shaped the book's logic and architecture so it would make sense and be friendlier to people without a medical background. I am most grateful for her help and sense of humor.

Dr. Sana Isa-Pratt is my personal physician and I am indebted to her for letting me (sometimes with trepidation) try new things: undertake weird experiments to become healthier, travel afar to seek medical wisdom, cleanse, fast, and generally experiment with my body and use it as a laboratory. I could not ask for a better doctor and coconspirator on my health journey.

ACKNOWLEDGMENTS

Several leading doctors, researchers, and health experts shared their expertise in personal interviews that were especially helpful in understanding specific habits and the latest ideas about how we approach our health and health care.

I am forever grateful to Becky Su, MD, EAMP, for her inspiration, patience, and passion to share her knowledge and healing with me and the world at large. A constant guide on my journey of health and the health habits shared in this book, Dr. Su founded and directs the Bellevue Acupuncture Clinic. Trained in Western medicine in China, Dr. Su is a master practitioner of acupuncture and traditional Chinese medicine who studied at Bastyr University in Kenmore, Washington, and serves on its board of trustees.

Julie Starkel, MS, MBA, RDN, is a leading holistically oriented nutritionist based in Seattle. The founder of Starkel Nutrition, she earned a master of science degree in whole foods clinical nutrition at Bastyr University and is a registered dietitian nutritionist and certified dietitian and a member of the Academy of Nutrition and Dietetics and the Institute for Functional Medicine. She thinks of nutrition as the foundation of all areas of health. Combining intellectual rigor, clarity, and a belief in the body's natural healing abilities, she brings the power of food to an integrative, functional approach to disease, healing, and wellness.

I am enormously grateful to Mimi Guarneri, MD, FACC, for her wisdom, research, and vision, which she so generously shared at a conference for health professionals and in a private interview for this book. She is changing the way medicine is practiced, how doctors approach their work, and how health is achieved. An inspiring and groundbreaking leader and author of *108 Pearls to Awaken Your Healing Potential,* she is president of the Academy of Integrative Health and Medicine and former president of the American Board of Integrative Holistic Medicine. Dr. Guarneri also served as senior advisor to the Atlantic Health System for the Chambers Center for Well Being. She is the founder and medical director of Guarneri Integrative Health, Inc., at Pacific Pearl La Jolla in California, and she founded the Scripps Center for Integrative Medicine where she served as medical director for 15 years.

We were fortunate to discover the work of Mark P. Mattson, PhD, during the research for this book and to get his firsthand insights in a personal interview. Dr. Mattson is a leading expert on intermittent fasting and the science that can help us understand the impact of our eating habits on our cellular and cognitive functions and reducing the risks of neurodegenerative diseases. Chief of the

Laboratory of Neurosciences at the National Institute on Aging and professor of neuroscience at Johns Hopkins University, his research and experiments with healthy eating in his own life have been an inspiration to me.

Another leap was needed to go from knowledge, experience, and stories to a form on the page that would speak to readers and inspire change. Janet Goldstein is a terrific writer, and her talents were paramount in creating this book. I am grateful for her insights and diligence as she helped me bring all the parts of *30 Summers More* to life. I also acknowledge the expertise of Aegis Living's Chief Marketing Officer Angie Snyder, editor Teddy Roberts, and my favorite creative genius, designer Jennifer Bartlett.

Many thanks to all of you,

Dwayne

Lessons From Longevity's Front Line

Just the other day, while commuting to work, I heard four science-based health stories on the radio: one on how a group of people with Parkinson's disease responded favorably to cycling three times a week; another on the reality that many drugs tested on mice don't work on people; a third on the question of the health benefits of marijuana; and finally, a report on why lonely people have more severe cold symptoms.

My daily ride to work takes less than 20 minutes.

We live in a fast-paced, information-rich age, yet there are many days when I try to learn more but end up understanding less about the very things that are important to me. The same is probably true for you, too!

One of my lifelong obsessions has been the pursuit of health—understanding it and attaining it. As a young kid, that meant I was an athlete and challenged my body's limits. After I became a young adult, I lost sight of that passion and I burned the proverbial candle at both ends. I worked long hours to start my career, ate my fill of junk food, often partied until dawn, and slept very little. I woke up the next morning just to repeat the cycle.

Although this is a common backstory, I have a personal plotline with details that diverge from the norm. For the past few decades, I've been an executive in the field of senior living. Many years ago, I founded my own elder care company, Aegis Living, which I still run today. In my several decades of proximity to the elderly, I have learned from the wisest and most simple, from the bravest and most adventuresome, from those impaired by hereditary diseases, from brilliant inventors and successful investors, and from the most loving and humble teachers, scholars, and public servants.

My back-of-the-napkin estimate is that I've overseen the care of more than 60,000 amazing human beings; and the stories I could tell. But those are for another time.

What is relevant for this book is that as I moved into my middle-age years, the psychic impact of my constant awareness of aging and death made me intensely curious about living a good life, and, even more, living the greatest life possible. Ironically, I'd never consciously applied those lessons to myself. I didn't think I needed them.

As I moved from my hard-charging 20s and 30s and into my 40s and early 50s, my health was increasingly going sideways. I made up a lot of stories about what I needed to do—for example, if I lost a few pounds and my clothes fit better, I'd be healthier and happier; if I worked out a bit harder at the gym, hammering my muscles, so my increased strength would make me look and feel healthier; if I took a few more medications, I could control the fates of illness and inevitable decline.

Oh boy! How could I be so smart and so dumb at the same time? I had bought into the myth that our health is an external thing—measured by how good we look and how functional we are—and not an internal process that maintains and transforms our health at a cellular level. (You won't doubt this fact after you read the first few chapters!)

One of the most important insights I discovered came from investigating our Western philosophy and system of health care. Many of our medical professionals are specialized and compartmentalized. The heart doctor doesn't know what the lung doctor is recommending, and neither doctor realizes that the kidney doctor has an entirely different approach that conflicts with their guidance. This specialization syndrome permeates so much of our lives, adding to our sense of being overwhelmed and confused. When so-called alternative approaches are added to the mix, taking care of ourselves becomes even more complicated.

Think about the last health-related self-help book you bought. I bet it was about a specific diet, new exercise routine, or proven approach to addressing a symptom or illness you're dealing with. However, these elements of health are not distinct from each other. They are all connected.

An argument can be made that our grandparents' era of taking care of ourselves was easier—fewer available choices caused fewer mistakes. Our modern lives are impacted by the abundance of everything, from virtually instant access and delivery of any consumer item on the planet to a continuous flow of information from family, friends, and the entire globe.

Our modern lives have also put the issue of civility front and center. Our poor sleep habits are making us cranky, and our daily food and exercise choices take our blood sugars on a mood-altering roller-coaster ride. This combination is making us very angry people, and we've lost the ability to be civil with one another. I believe if we pay more attention to our health, perhaps we could reduce the anger and meanness and bring civility back into our lives.

We cannot—nor should we want to—reverse time and limit our incredibly exciting modern lives. Nonetheless, as aware as we are, I've found there's one basic, timeless goal for everyone I talk with about health and longevity. Most people want to live well, live to an acceptable, relatively healthy old age (funny how everyone has a different number), and then die happily in their sleep one night with no burdensome suffering.

You may not be able to script how you die, but you can adopt habits that will make it much more likely that you live well, age in healthier ways, and improve the quality of your life in your middle and final chapters. If you take away just one thing from this book, it'll be this: *know that you have the power to change your health destiny right now.* I've learned it and I live it.

The title *30 Summers More* was inspired by a conversation with a good friend. We were sitting on a beach on Whidbey Island, looking out over the water as the sun began to set. It was warm, the landscape breathtaking, our conversation deep. We discussed the limited time all of us have on the planet, and whether we are making the most of our time here. If we have only 30 of these glorious Pacific Northwest summers left, what will we do and how will we make sure we are healthy enough to enjoy them?

My answer about aging healthfully is to practice the life-giving behaviors detailed in this book. I hope it challenges your thinking and inspires your actions around your health. I want to share the strategies I've learned that can literally change your life, which is possible if you take charge of your own health. I hope you find just one or two gold nuggets—or maybe many more—in this book and make use of them.

So, let's begin the journey together.

Waking Up

Understanding Our True Health Potential— Now and As We Age

Like a lot of people, I didn't do so well by my body for a long time, even though I tried—and even though I'd been a leader in helping older people with their health and wellness for more than 30 years.

I'm sure some of you reading this book have amazing diets, exercise routines, meditation practices, holistic remedies, and medical histories. I can bet that few of you, however, are living a life that maximizes your health potential. I've learned that these beliefs are widely shared:

- We want longer and better-quality lives, but we worry there's little we can do to stay healthy and mentally sharp as we age.

- We want quick fixes, and those rarely work and often backfire. We end up with sports injuries, medical side effects, and disappointment in ourselves when we don't meet our expectations.

- We want there to be a cost benefits to making changes—especially the ones that makes us look good on the outside, no matter what's happening on the inside.

- We want an "edge" in thriving into old age, but we're overwhelmed by advice. We become obsessed with perfection, defeating the purpose of healthy living, or we throw up our hands and tell ourselves it's not worth pursuing.

What I see are too many people giving in to midlife—giving in to the moment when they don't feel young anymore, when they are achy and are tired, don't recovery as quickly, panic with the arrival of memory gaps, and have more and more complaints.

Of course, many people *seem* to be doing great: they're at the peak of their careers, have rewarding relationships, and may be seeing their children coming into successful adulthood. Be that as it may, peak potential is rarely showing up in how they care for themselves and how they feel. A famous quote by the Dalai Lama says it best. When asked what surprised him most about humanity, he said,

Man. Because he sacrifices his health in order to make money. Then he sacrifices money to recuperate his health. And then he is so anxious about the future that he does not enjoy the present; the result being that he does not live in the present or the future; he lives as if he is never going to die, and then dies having never really lived.

The Japanese concept of *karoshi* comes to mind when I think of what can happen when you aren't in tune with your body's needs. *Karoshi,* a Japanese word that literally translates as "overwork death," is known as sudden occupational mortality. In South Korea it's called *gwarosa* and in China, *guolaosi.* The term is said to have originated in 1982 when three Japanese doctors published a book about *karoshi* that noted many victims of overwork and included research into their deaths. The victims were young men who were otherwise healthy but had worked more than 60 hours a week on average and had died on the job from heart attacks and strokes. There are reports that as many as 10,000 people a year die from *karoshi* and many are in their 20s.

Karoshi also is acknowledged in the United States, so I bring this up as a reminder for you to check in with your body often and stay in tune with it, especially if you are a workaholic. Overworking is no laughing matter and can be detrimental to your health, even fatal. The old adage that hard work never killed anyone is certainly incorrect.

The Hand We're Dealt—And the Hand We Create

I've been overweight all my life, but I've always been active—earlier as an athlete in school and later with workouts. Then everything started catching up with me. I felt like I was falling off a cliff.

I had grown up poor—though rich in my mother's dreams for me—and felt driven to succeed. Success meant financial security and the lifestyle I thought I deserved. Even though I indulged, when I looked at my parents and saw how well they were aging, I thought, "I've inherited their genes and they lived long lives, so I guess I'm lucky and I will too." (You would be surprised how many people think this.)

What I didn't realize was that my parents spent their lifetimes being much more active and eating more healthfully than I did. They ate fresh foods—some grown in their garden—and prepared them at home. They overcame the stress of their challenging early years and the breakup of their marriage. Each in their own way appreciated what they had, their friends, and the communities they'd settled in.

When I think about how much more natural movement my parents had in their lives, the iPhone comes to mind. This minicomputer, a butler in a way, eliminated the need for us to move like people one or two generations before us. For example, today we don't get up to answer the phone, go to the encyclopedia, shop in a store, or get out of the chair to change the channel on the television.

Speaking of television, while researching this book I found that frozen TV dinners were introduced in 1954 and rocketed in popularity, intentionally drawing people away from eating dinner at the table. This helped create some of the eating problems we have today. Moving into the 1960s, Western food science brought us toaster pastries, sugary cereals, and cheese-flavored tortilla chips all dressed up in attention-grabbing packaging. The 1970s gave us frozen waffles. You get the idea: unhealthy. Tasty food got fast, cheap, and easy. In my opinion, these changes to our food and the decrease in our natural movement began a culture of gluttony.

> I SEE TOO MANY PEOPLE GIVING IN TO MIDLIFE. GIVING IN TO THE MOMENT WHEN THEY DON'T FEEL YOUNG ANYMORE.

My parents were not raised in this gluttonous culture. Their generation rationed and budgeted for everything, including food, water, soap, and clothing. Today, we have this gift of access to so much food no matter what the season. Unfortunately, this gift has developed to a point that it hurts us.

What I see today is almost like an Armageddon. I see my generation and others not realizing that this easy access to food and technology is shortening our lives—but we don't have to let it. We can benefit from a more disciplined approach to our eating habits and natural movement.

In fact, as a little boy I remember my grandmother telling me what she called "the sweet story" from her childhood, before the turn of the 20th century, back when savoring one sweet treat could provide days of pleasure.

My grandmother's father would go to the store and buy her one sweet, a piece of rock candy. On Saturday, he would give it to her wrapped in wax paper and would tell her she could have three swirls—three licks with her tongue. Then he'd have her put the candy back in its wax paper until the next Saturday, when he'd give it to her again. My grandmother said that one sweet would last two months.

My life was so different. I indulged and thought it was my due. I had a health scare at 34—a bleeding ulcer. I was told if I didn't change my diet I would have major problems later in life, but I ignored the warning. I loved fast food and rich dinners, and I ate way too much. There seemed no way around it. I was the typical meat-and-potatoes guy who wouldn't pass up a large rib eye steak.

As I progressed in my career, although I consistently went to the gym three to four days a week, I no longer mowed my lawn, washed my car, did my laundry, or even walked my dog. My parents, however, having none of the help I did, were on the move most of the day.

My father died when I was 49 and he was 84½ years old. I went to his home two days after he was found deceased. His nephew, whose farm he lived on, showed me a trench that was 35 feet long and four feet wide. I have no idea what it was for, but this old man, who still smoked two packs of unfiltered cigarettes a day, had dug it the day before he died. I was amazed.

As I entered my 40s, my weight began to soar. Within a couple of years, I'd gained almost 40 pounds and hit an all-time high body weight. My goal of building a company and achieving wealth had a perverse effect on my health. I found myself on the "pill cure": a pill for this, a pill for that. Lots of my friends were in similar situations. They started finding themselves on statins and heart medicine when they hit the big five-oh or six-oh.

In my case, I was taking blood pressure pills, antacids, cholesterol meds, steroids, and inhalers for my asthma, which wasn't under control. When I suffered a bout of gout with painful inflammation in my foot, I was miserable.

My Wake-Up Call

Everything came to a head after a particularly fabulous Labor Day weekend with my wife, T. It was an Aegis senior staff weekend where we worked hard during the planned schedule of meetings and played hard in between. I wanted to keep up with the younger people, so there I was, lifting weights in the gym, participating in every strenuous activity offered, and popping ibuprofen to prepare for the inevitable soreness.

In the downtime, T and I enjoyed the outdoors and sunshine—a treat in overcast Seattle—while at the same time I binged on sweet goodies laid out for the weekend. Out of the blue—well, it wasn't out of the blue, but it seemed that way—I had the most acute abdominal pain I'd ever experienced. It was so bad that I ended up in the hospital and was eventually diagnosed with severe gastritis.

All the ibuprofen I'd taken had acted like acid in my colon, which was already stressed from the health issues with which I was struggling. The medical team couldn't stop the bleeding for two days. I was terrified. The doctors were close to giving me a blood transfusion. I asked them to hold off for a day, which everyone felt was reasonable, and gradually my body started to stabilize.

I was in the hospital for a couple of days, physically and emotionally shaken up. I sent my mind to my higher power and knew that I needed to start a new journey. I knew that I had a choice. I could wake up. I wasn't going to make it to 80—surely not in a healthy, independent state—if I didn't change how I was living and caring for myself.

As I sat in my hospital bed, I ruminated on the manuscript I'd begun that was sitting at home on my desk. I asked T to bring me the pages—there was nothing else to occupy me in my condition.

As I read, I saw right away that while I'd been living and breathing questions about the health and longevity of the residents of Aegis, I'd separated myself from what I'd learned. Overnight, my commitment changed. I was no longer working on a book about longevity. I had to pivot to a focus on healthy living—in our 50s, 60s, and even 70s. I felt that in a way, maybe this health crisis was given to me in a way so I would pursue longevity, learn even more about it, and share my knowledge with a broader audience to help them. So it was a turning point for the book and an even bigger one for me.

Investigating Healthy Longevity: Four Principles That Are the Foundation of My Experiences

I wanted to understand the intertwined strands of luck, fate, genes, and habits. I wanted to know which aspects of longevity were a given and which were ours for the taking. In other words, what could I do that would give me a healthy edge? What really keeps us well? What were the root causes leading me and others to get sick? And what was *really* killing us?

I'm not a scientist, but I began an intensive investigation. I read books, lay articles, and scientific papers. I discussed, debated, and further dug into the biology and science of health and aging with Shirley Newell, MD, Aegis Living's passionate and compassionate chief medical officer. We also sent our researcher back out to research even more journals and reports.

At the same time, I spent hundreds of hours in conversations with health experts and ordinary people. I talked to friends and colleagues, doctors, laboratory scientists, my massage therapist, and dozens of Aegis residents and other 80-, 90-, and 100-year-olds—all in an effort to better understand the overwhelming amount of information and advice out there and understand what is doable for most of us. I also drew on my experiences traveling to many of the countries ranked highest in health and well-being by the World Health Organization, from France and Italy to Japan and Singapore. (That's my favorite kind of "study"—the serendipity of meeting people, hearing their stories, and gaining small tidbits of advice.)

From all this exploration, four foundational premises rose to the surface and became the underlying message of this book: *we're not stuck with our current level of health and happiness.*

These are the premises:

1. **Genetics.** These play a much smaller part in our health and longevity than most of us believe. Depending on the study, 65% to 80% of our health and wellness is within our control. We're not at the mercy of our genes. Our genetic inheritance—that is, the expression of our genes—is not fixed. It can change, depending on factors we can control. Although we can't guarantee our destiny, a large part of it is in our own hands.

2. **Cells.** Our bodies are made up of cells, which are renewing and wearing out in a complex dance affected by our underlying health, habits, and environment. Our cells are continually generating, dying, and regenerating, and their healthy life span is significantly in our control. Everything we do either contributes to the preservation or destruction of our cells. The process of cell death can be slowed down, and sometimes cells can be rejuvenated. Some years ago, this notion may have seemed like science fiction. But today it is an observable fact. Our choices have a tangible impact on the health and longevity of our cells.

> WE'RE NOT STUCK WITH OUR CURRENT LEVEL OF HEALTH AND HAPPINESS. NO MATTER OUR AGE OR CURRENT SITUATION, MOST OF US CAN BE HEALTHIER LONGER.

3. **Inflammation.** A largely hidden or overlooked root cause of illness, inflammation in the body cuts too many lives short. This premise is the one that has shaped my own attitudes and personal actions most profoundly. According to the United States Centers for Disease Control and Prevention, the five leading causes of death in America, excluding accidental death, are, in order, cancer, lower respiratory disease, stroke, Alzheimer's disease, and diabetes. These devastating illnesses have one thing in common: they all are inflammatory. If we want to minimize the things that are killing us, we need to reduce the inflammation of our cells, which is doable!

4. **Health habits.** We can significantly increase our health during our middle and later years through our choices—our habits of health. That's five years of cognitive, physical, and emotional wellness that can change our lives. We now know that aging is hardwired in our cells, but our cellular life spans are not fixed. Although it's true that all of us are at increased risk for Alzheimer's and cancer simply by getting older, our habits of health can improve our odds of avoiding or delaying the onset of some diseases.

One recent national life expectancy study showed that even the health risks of poverty, which are closely associated with earlier death, could be lessened by the simple habit of walking. I was amazed to learn that walking added some six years to lives of the lowest-income residents in New York City—known as a walking city—because people must walk to shops, subways, and buses to get around rather than relying on cars. In spite of factors such as poor diet, high levels of stress, and exposure to pollution, walking (along with some public health initiatives) protected the health and extended life spans of a whole population.

Habits of Health

I learned that every single one of our healthy habits—from walking to sleeping to eating—supports and extends the life of our cells and has the capacity to improve our brain function, heart and gut health, mental equilibrium, the inflammation that affects so much of our well-being, and our resilience. No matter what our age or current situation, most of us can be healthier longer, even if we are dealing with an illness or a chronic condition.

The path to health that I created for myself is made of seven habits:

1. **Wellness:** Taking control of your own health—and believing it matters—makes all the rest of the habits possible.

2. **Health knowledge:** Understanding the cellular basis of health and having curiosity about how your body functions can give you powerful insights and the incentive to make better choices. It also contributes to a sense of purpose and happiness.

3. **Eating:** You don't have to be overwhelmed. The basics of a healthy approach to eating can fit in a chapter! If you are dealing with specific issues, you can layer on additional targeted and personalized approaches.

4. **Moving:** "Exercising" is not enough and can be misguided. We need a new message about movement in our lives to counter today's life-sapping lifestyle of sitting.

5. **Sleeping:** We can't function well if we don't rest. Lack of sufficient or deep sleep is often a silent factor that disrupts your total health, including your eating, your heart health, your digestion and gut problems, your mood, and so much more.

6. **Relationships:** A good marriage goes a long way for longevity, and having deep, happy relationships with friends is a powerful antioxidant for your body and emotional well-being.

7. **Purpose:** Having a purpose in life—a reason to get up every day—leads to happiness and a sense of meaning. Becoming aware of the interconnectedness of your physical and emotional health can strengthen your mood and resilience, relationships, ability to manage stress, and daily sense of joy.

One Step at a Time

I wish I could say I've become a poster child for healthy living. I haven't, but I have increased my healthy behaviors and eliminated a lot of risks by slowing down, doing just a bit less, and trying at all costs not to blow off time with family and friends because of work. I'm giving my body and mind more time to rest and recharge.

I've lost 50 pounds since my time in the hospital and these pounds are not coming back. I've given up most dairy and sugar and reduced my caloric intake. I get regular acupuncture and reflexology treatments, and I do qigong or tai chi a few times a week in addition to my gym workouts. I walk more and I'm sleeping better than ever. Transcendental meditation is something I've incorporated into my routine, and it's had a profound effect for me. All these practices have improved my energy, and I feel better—I feel well.

I've taken charge of my own health, and it feels good. I've gone from being on medication for asthma, high cholesterol, and high blood sugar to very few. The reason? The health habits I cover in this book significantly decrease inflammation in the body, which in turn prevents five of the most common inflammation-based diseases we face today—Alzheimer's disease, arthritis, asthma, diabetes, and heart disease.

From my personal experience, I can tell you that these habits of health are not a struggle when your metabolism is in balance, your inflammation is reduced, and your heart is no longer racing. The habits you'll learn in this book have helped me have a substantially better quality of life, and I know that they'll help you, too.

Your Turn to Wake Up

So it's your turn. The things I've done, maybe you don't want to do all of them, but I'm betting that you will find a few of them easy and enjoyable. Start with one and layer things in bit by bit. Remember: it's not one or two big habits, it's the many microhabits we develop that help us live well. I've listed all my microhabits throughout the book and at the end as a list. Yours might be different from mine, but mine can give you a start.

Imagine your next week, month, year, and decade. Think about your path to finding your healthy edge—that place where your habits of health lead to greater energy, stamina, and ease—with the health numbers to match. Experiment with the simple yet powerful recommendations in this book—or wherever you find them. Be well. Recover well. Live well. Share your journey with the people who matter most to you.

A Simple Self-Assessment

What's your current health story?

Arriving at mid- and later life, we all have a set of conscious and unconscious beliefs about our health and what it means to live the good life. I've shared my story and beliefs with you. Now it's your turn to reflect on yours. Take a few minutes now to see where you are. Write in this book or start your own health journal, and I encourage you to take notes as you read this book. If the process of writing and sharing the ideas in here is any guide, each of you will find different habits, insights, bits of inspiration, and practical strategies that speak to your needs and personalities. We'll talk more about tracking your habits, but for now, start where you are.

What practices do you have in place now to improve your health and wellness?
This includes activities such as moving your body, learning about health, eating well, and avoiding specific foods.

_____

_____

_____

_____

_____

_____

_____

_____

_____

How many hours a day do these activities take?

_____

_____

_____

_____

_____

_____

Name the ways you stay in tune with the condition of your body. Do you weigh yourself daily, take your own blood pressure and check your blood sugar, or journal how you feel each day?

_____

_____

_____

_____

_____

_____

Sit with your eyes closed and ask yourself a simple question: What is giving me pain or discomfort? Give your body permission to tell you all the areas that are affected. Wait for each area to report in as you mentally scan your body, then write them down one by one. You will be shocked by what you may not have been fully conscious of before.

_____

_____

_____

_____

_____

_____

What kinds of foods make your body react negatively, and what is the specific reaction? For example, dairy might make you feel nauseated, or you may feel tired after you eat pancakes with syrup.

_____

_____

_____

_____

_____

_____

How many minutes do you spend eating each meal?

Breakfast _____

Lunch _____

Dinner _____

List the ways you get natural movement in your day, and estimate how many of these steps make up your daily step total. This includes household chores, walking around the grocery store or at work, or working in the garden.

_____

_____

_____

_____

_____

_____

_____

_____

_____

_____

_____

How do you work on your balance, and how often do you do it? For example, do you practice yoga, tai chi, or standing on one foot while brushing your teeth?

_____

_____

_____

_____

_____

_____

Do you sleep well? Describe your nightly routine during the two hours before you go to bed. Rapid eye movement (REM) and deep sleep should be about 1.5 hours or more of your total night's sleep.

_____

_____

_____

_____

_____

_____

_____

_____

How is your bedroom conducive to a good night's sleep? Do you have bedding that is comfortable, is the temperature of the room cool at night, and is it quiet?

_____

_____

_____

_____

_____

_____

How many close relationships do you have? How do you nurture them? See if you can name three people other than your spouse.

_____

_____

_____

_____

_____

_____

How do you describe your life purpose? There is no wrong answer, but it should be something that would get you up every morning and let you know you are needed. Examples include playing with your grandkids three days a week, working on an environmental or political cause, or spreading the word about a subject you care about.

_____

_____

_____

_____

_____

_____

_____

_____

_____

_____

_____

_____

_____

Know Thyself

TAKE CHARGE OF YOUR HEALTH AND HEALTH CARE

"Each patient carries his own doctor inside him.
They come to us now knowing this truth.
We are at our best when they give the doctor
who resides within each patient
a chance to go to work."

—ALBERT SCHWEITZER,
MISSIONARY SURGEON, HUMANITARIAN, AND NOBEL LAUREATE

Your good health requires a strong captain, and that's you. I learned that the best way to be one is to focus on prevention, be proactive about my own well-being, and remember that simple changes can make a big difference. Inside this chapter I'll show you that:

- To stay well, you must become a partner with your doctor in caring for your body. A great way to do this is to document your baseline health numbers daily.

- When you go prepared to a doctor appointment, your doctor may spend more of your precious appointment time accurately diagnosing and treating you, rather than assessing you.

- Carefully choosing your medical practitioners is essential to good health.

- Our Western model of medicine is broken. To help compensate, look for an integrative medical practitioner who will analyze your entire health story and work to solve the root causes of your health challenges, rather than just ease symptoms.

- Self-awareness is extremely important. Just because you look great doesn't mean you are in great health.

- You deserve to have the right doctor for you and to question medical practitioners if you don't understand what they told you or if something doesn't seem "quite right."

Picture the shore of a lake or ocean where someone has pushed a stick into the sand. The stick stands straight up, supported by a mound of sand piled up around it. If that stick starts to lean to one side, you can prop it up by reinforcing the pile of sand at its base. Over time, the waves and wind will scoop away some of the sand. Without intervention, a little more sand will wash away, and then a little more, until the stick is about to topple over.

Your body is like that stick—sturdy but vulnerable. If you don't take care of your body, or if you ignore the signs that its foundation—your health—is compromised, you'll have a problem. When we don't support our bodies with healthy habits, we're wearing our bodies down. There is no stasis. We're either strengthening our health or weakening it.

Dr. Becky Su, a brilliant practitioner of Western and Chinese medicine, introduced me to the sandpile metaphor. She has been a healing presence—and friend—in my own life and has helped me learn how to actively strengthen my body and health.

Ownership of Our Health Means *Partnership*

Traditionally, we didn't look to ourselves to ensure our health. We looked to our doctors. Whenever my mother went to the doctor, she put on her best suit and lipstick and saw the appointment as time for a bit of flirting, as if she were meeting her heartthrob Cary Grant. (The doctors always were male.) Whatever the doctor said, her response was "yes, sir" or "no, sir."

But gone are the days when we can think of our doctors as the authorities who tell us exactly which tests, medicines, and procedures to have. Doctors and patients alike are bombarded with new information and treatment options, and our care providers seem to be busier than ever. That means you need to be a proactive, informed partner. The goal is not to replace our doctors; the goal is to become our own best medical advocates and personal medical historians.

I track my health numbers daily. I want to know my trends so I can help my doctors spend less of their limited time assessing me, and more time diagnosing and treating me. For example, one year I noticed that my blood pressure was creeping up. I was doing all the things I know to do to keep it down. On my own I'd even added testosterone to my regimen to increase my well-being. I took my baseline blood pressure readings into Dr. Su, and right away she said that the testosterone was the likely culprit. She explained that adding testosterone to a 57-year-old body is like putting a new race car engine into a Studebaker. The engine is new, but all the other car parts are much older and cannot keep up with the engine. In my case, the testosterone could have given me a heart attack.

For most of us, monitoring and tracking our bodies constitutes a paradigm shift. Yet you know your body and how you feel better than anyone else does. You know the baseline for what's normal and healthy for you and what's not. You're the only one who can say, "I feel better." Yes, it takes some investigation, work, and education, but when you take charge of your own health, you help your doctor help you.

Your doctor is likely to spend an average of 12 to 18 minutes with you during the average office visit. That's the truth. Of course, there are times when your doctor might spend 45 minutes or an hour with you, but the time constraints are real. You can be angry at the medical system, or you can flip your mind-set and become an active participant.

Think about it this way. How many times have you gone to the doctor for an annual checkup, and when asked how you're feeling, you say, "Everything is fine?" Or, when you're being treated for an illness, how many times have you underplayed your symptoms of discomfort or pain? A friend of mine recently told me that the nicest thing a doctor ever told her was, "You look terrible." It made her feel that the doctor understood and would truly help.

Always go into your doctor appointment prepared. I get ready for mine like I do for a business meeting. I don't wait for the doc to ask me questions. I hand over my health log with all my numbers and tell the doc what is going on right away—*here's my baseline, my fever was X, my pain is at a seven.* Help your doctor get to the conclusions. Ninety percent of her or his job is assessment, but because I track my health, my doctors can get right to diagnosis and treatment. That is how to help your doc help you the best. When I go to my doctor with my notes and charts in hand, I know that she thinks, "Wow, I need to pay attention. This isn't ordinary for Dwayne. Something is going on."

We are so very different and it's why your active input is required. Being a participant in your health means understanding your own body. For example, I don't think I could ever be a vegetarian. I can't eat dairy. I tell this to practitioners who are new to me to ensure that they work with me in recommending dietary adjustments.

Choose Your Doctors Carefully

Your doctors have a specific level of medical knowledge, and they of course play an important role in your health. However, just because they have the credentials doesn't mean you should give them a pass from careful scrutiny before they diagnose, prescribe, or operate on you. You know when you are off-kilter, and understand the severity and magnitude of your issue.

We spend more time shopping for the right phone or laptop than we do shopping for the right doctor. It's crazy to go in and blindly trust a surgeon you've met once to stick a knife in you. Check out reports on ethics, malpractice, and any litigation that may be pending. Author of the book *Outliers* and journalist for *The New Yorker* Malcolm Gladwell states that it takes 10,000 hours of practice to achieve mastery in a field. Personally, I want the doc who adheres to this theory and has done the procedure 10,000 times—unless of course the procedure is rare and this isn't possible. Either way, you want an expert, so do the due diligence. I mean, talk about a way to increase longevity!

In 2016, Martin Makary, a professor of surgery at the Johns Hopkins School of Medicine, led a research study that identified medical errors as the third leading cause of death in the United States. That's 251,454 people annually. Why isn't this commonly known? The Centers for Disease Control and Prevention doesn't collect this information because the medical billing codes it tracks don't include a code for death by medical error.

An Evolving Understanding of Cures and the Role of Habits

The nature of health at midlife and beyond has changed. Many diseases—even some cancers—are becoming chronic conditions that we can treat and sometimes live with into old age.

> A BIG PART OF BEING WELL MEANS TAKING CHARGE AND BELIEVING THAT SIMPLE CHANGES MAKE A TANGIBLE DIFFERENCE.

A 2016 article in the *New York Times* called "We Won't Cure Cancer" by Jarle Breivik, MD, PhD, a professor of medicine at the Institute of Basic Medical Sciences at the University of Oslo, explained that cancer is a condition of our aging cells. As we live longer, he says our cells are "more prone to going astray." However, that's not the end of the story. Breivik concluded his article with a powerful, optimistic message: although cancer research is producing astonishing science, leading to new treatments and cures, many more lives can be saved by doing the boring stuff, such as getting people to stop smoking, eat healthfully, exercise, and put on sunscreen.

Many people are trained to quickly reach for medication when we aren't feeling quite right. We cheat our body's natural healing abilities and become dependent on artificial means to make us feel better. Instead, try this simple formula:

1. **Hydration.** I drink a glass of room temperature water upon waking and a good deal of water throughout the day.

2. **Meditation.** Twenty minutes twice a day of transcendental meditation works for me.

3. **Medication.** If you still are not feeling quite right, then try medication, but I think you will be shocked at how hydration and meditation will rebalance your body.

In addition, getting more and better sleep, consciously taking care of our emotions and relationships, and maintaining a lifelong sense of purpose are important. These are the habits that affect our health and the longevity of our cells.

Developing a wellness habit means taking charge and believing that simple changes make a tangible difference. Looking for miracle pills, cures, and elixirs misses a bigger truth: even if you're a cancer survivor, even if you've experienced a heart attack or a stroke or have an ongoing medical condition, the healthy choices you start making—or intensifying—can affect your life now and your health and happiness in the months and years ahead.

Science is proving the miracle that many of us are missing: the benefits that come from healthy habits and meaningful, simple living that so many of our grandparents enjoyed. The aggregate benefits are huge.

Attitudes Affect Our Actions

Wellness isn't only an intellectual idea—it's an emotional and psychological one, too. Wellness has to do with our beliefs.

Too many people define *getting older* not as *aging* but as *declining*. This leads us to (1) ignore the changes of aging or (2) succumb to them and just give up.

Ignoring these changes can lead us to act like 30-year-olds with the potential for danger everywhere. I have a number of CEO friends who are extreme adventurers. They want me to do crazy things with them—jump out of airplanes; climb the tallest mountain peaks; go heli-skiing. I tell them that I wouldn't make it out of the bus to the starting location.

You need to be practical about who you are and know your health limits. At the same time, you want to stretch yourself. I'm not going to run a marathon, but I'll lift moderate weights that would be too taxing for many people. I'll go on hikes, exercise at the gym, swim, and try new things in tune with my health.

The other side is succumbing to the changes. If your mind tells you that the negative effects of aging are inevitable, you're predisposed to accept limitations and incapacity rather than pursue your potential for extended and even improved health. I want to encourage you to remove those limiting beliefs. If your doctor says you've got a clean bill of health, you can maintain an active, adventurous life consistent with your personal limits.

I love this case in point: On a ski vacation in Sun Valley, I stepped into a small shop to pick out a gift for my wife. The woman who came over to help me seemed like a really sweet older lady. As I looked at various items, we got to chatting, and I asked if she'd ever skied. To my astonishment, she answered that she started skiing in the 1950s. So of course I had to ask if she still skied. She said,

"Oh sure. In fact, I'm in a race tomorrow."

"A race?" I said.

"Yeah, I'm a downhill racer."

She had raced in Sun Valley for years, and at 84 years old, was involved in senior ski competitions, and had been in an Olympics qualifier. She got a kick out of telling me about the old-timer guys who wore skintight gear with their tummies sticking out.

When I asked her if she'd ever been hurt, she paused for a minute and then answered, "You know, I broke a thumb in the '60s"

Here's a woman living at her healthy edge. If you have high blood pressure or heart disease, then don't go racing on the slopes. Put yourself on the health scale and be responsible, but don't succumb to limits in your head.

Don't Underestimate the Power of Awareness

Let's say that you're basically healthy and you rate yourself a seven on a scale of one to ten. Now, let's say you get a cold and your immune system gets busy fighting it off. A week later, your body is more susceptible than usual and you get the flu, which lasts four days. You think you're over it and decide to return to your workout routine, and this adds another stressor to your system. That night you go out with friends and have four glasses of wine and don't sleep well. You wake up groggy, your blood pressure goes up, and that night you pull an all-nighter to finish a big report for work. Or, if you skip the all-nighter, you might take a sleeping pill or cold medicine to knock yourself out, causing a negative effect on your still-depleted immune system. A lack of awareness about the layer after punishing layer your body is absorbing can become quite dangerous.

If you have any underlying weaknesses, you're now at greater risk for a major event such as a heart attack or stroke. If you were to end up in the emergency room, people might say, "My God, what happened? Last year you ran a half marathon!" It's extremely rare, however, to have a major medical issue that just happens out of the blue. Like my Labor Day gastritis emergency when I had an accumulation of signs, almost always there's a trend of changes. Those are the signs that we try to ignore and may hide from the people who care about us. If we don't adjust, it's a bit like driving a car 150 mile per hour on a track without measuring our gauges—that's an accident waiting to happen unless you're driving a car with the right setup.

If you're driving down a highway and your dashboard warning light shows that something is wrong and your gas tank is low, you wouldn't drive 150 miles an hour. You'd maintain a steady 50 miles an hour as you headed to the nearest gas station. When it comes to our bodies, however, too many of us ignore the signs, keeping up a pace that increases our risk of breakdown.

There's a health "muscle" you can't overdevelop, though: awareness. You can become aware of your body and your preconceived ideas about your health.

A Broken Model: The Limits of Traditional Western Health Care

Being proactive means shifting your beliefs and partnering with your doctors, and it also means taking a broader view of health—one that goes beyond the limiting perspective of Western medicine, which often is reactive and problem-focused rather than proactive and prevention-focused.

Mimi Guarneri, MD, president of the Academy of Integrative Health and Medicine and medical director of Guarneri Integrative Health in La Jolla, California, is one of the world's leading cardiologists and a healer to the very marrow of her bones. Searching for a better way to help her patients, she trained to become one of the world's leading integrative medicine experts, meaning the practice of health care that sees health as more than the absence of disease, and prevention as the best intervention. Dr. Guarneri explains:

> *Western medicine takes care of people after they break down and after they get sick. When someone has a disease, a chronic disease, like diabetes or heart disease or hypertension, Western medicine focuses on the "ill-to-the-pill" approach. For your diabetes, we give you this pill; for your hypertension, we give you that pill; for your heart disease, we give you this pill. The reality is that we never get to the underlying cause of the problem.*
>
> *After genetics, how we live our lives—the environment we live in, our daily approach to living—really is the determinant of our health. And even with our genes, we know they are not our destiny. Our genes require an environment in which to interact. But we don't focus on the environment and the underlying cause of our illnesses.*

We are good at translating the science of disease into practice, but
we're not good at translating the science of health into practice.

I've experienced the impact of this approach with my own health. Dr. Guarneri cites the proof demonstrated in many large-scale studies. For example, the 2004 INTERHEART study looked to 52 countries to answer this question: what leads to a heart attack?

As you might surmise from what you've read so far, the answers largely have to do with two factors: people's habits (tobacco use, sedentary lifestyle, unhealthy diet, and negative responses to stress and tension) and the conditions associated with those habits (obesity, abnormal lipids—fats and cholesterol).

The risk factors that cause lifestyle-related illnesses such as heart disease are the same as the risk factors that cause dementia and arthritis. If I'm obese and diabetic and not exercising, I'm probably going to have high blood pressure. There's also a good chance I'm at greater risk of experiencing memory loss and potentially Alzheimer's disease.

Likewise, there are the positive effects of healthy lifestyle factors. Dr. Guarneri points to the some 1,400 studies on the impact of eating a Mediterranean diet, which may reduce the development of cardiovascular events by 33% to 38%.

> "WE ARE GOOD AT TRANSLATING THE SCIENCE OF DISEASE INTO PRACTICE, BUT WE'RE NOT GOOD AT TRANSLATING THE SCIENCE OF HEALTH INTO PRACTICE."
>
> — Dr. Mimi Guarneri

Then there's the HALE project, which has looked at lifestyle changes in seven European countries and has concluded that it may be beneficial to start at any age. One aspect of the study evaluated people between the ages of 70 and 90 who made lifestyle changes and discovered that their new habits led to a 50% reduction in all-cause and cause-specific mortality.

Meditation, which is accessible to everyone, also has enormous potential for fostering wellness. According to Dr. Guarneri, "Transcendental Meditation reduces heart attack, stroke, and sudden death by 48%. That's better than any medicine I know."

In fact, I added Transcendental Meditation (also known as TM) to my list of habits to prevent illness and promote good health before publishing this book.

TM is part of the Vedic tradition of India, dating back thousands of years, and is a key element of Ayurveda (the science of life), one of the world's oldest systems of health care and personal development. The Transcendental Meditation movement originated with Maharishi Mahesh Yogi, founder of the organization, and continues on today after his death in 2008.

TM has been life changing for me. I do it twice a day for 20 minutes. It clears my brain of stress and distracting thoughts, it takes my blood pressure and blood sugar down, and I find that I have much more energy, clarity, and creativity now that it's part of my daily routine.

This form of meditation must be done twice a day for 20 minutes per meditation period. I have a packed schedule and finding two 20-minute blocks of time each day can be a challenge, but I do it. Even if it means I'm doing TM in the airport, in the back of a car, or a restaurant, I do it. It's not something you can do once in a while and expect results, but if you do it regularly, the time spent has an immediate return.

Other people also have positive things to say about the benefits of TM. Jerry Seinfeld, Liv Tyler, and Anderson Cooper are fans, too. However, the science speaks the loudest. According to a 2017 *Seattle Times* article on the subject, the most cited medical research on TM "is a 1989 Stanford University study that found TM is twice as effective at reducing anxiety when compared with concentration, contemplation and other techniques like deep breathing. Moreover, the American Medical Association released a study that shows TM reduces high blood pressure and mortality rates by almost 50% for those who have practiced for more than five years." So please, stop thinking about it and start doing it. What medication do you know of that can produce those results?

According to the David Lynch Foundation, the National Institutes of Health granted $26 million to several organizations to study the effects of TM on cardiovascular disease. These research findings mirror the information above because they found that TM:

- Decreases the incidence of heart attack, stroke, and death.
- Reduces the presence of metabolic syndrome.
- Extends longevity.
- Reduces blood pressure and use of hypertensive medications.
- Reduces constriction of blood vessels.

In short, TM is a wonderful health improvement habit to develop.

So back to my overarching point. Although our health care system excels in "sickness care" that identifies, diagnoses, and treats diseases, it frequently falls short of the goals of prevention. It also falls short with palliative care, which we can think of as the right care adapted to the desires, health status, and medical options for the patient. In other words, the needs of a young person will be different from the needs of an elderly, end-of-life patient.

For our purposes, if we want to take charge of our health, we have to think more broadly about health. Practitioners of integrative and functional medicine complement Western medicine with alternative approaches. They look at our bodies and health holistically, not as silos of body parts and conditions.

Dr. Becky Su came to her integrative approach to medicine through her own healing journey. Raised in China, she was sick all the time as a child and realized early on that she would have to become a doctor if she had any hope of being well. No one else would save her, she determined.

Dr. Su studied Western medicine and became an MD, but she continued to suffer from pain and overwork. One day, in the middle of performing surgery in the crowded Chinese hospital where she practiced, Dr. Su was overcome with terrible menstrual cramps. A nurse raced her over to an acupuncturist in the clinic. Those four acupuncture needles worked so well that she went back and finished the surgery she started. The experience also launched her interest in traditional Chinese medicine and acupuncture.

Eventually, Dr. Su was able to come to America and became a master practitioner of acupuncture and traditional Chinese medicine. This is how she sees the different approaches to health: "Treatment is good. Prevention is better. Empowering the body's healing power is superior."

When healthy habits are an integral part of your life, you improve your body's natural healing powers day to day. Then, you can draw on them when your body is facing a challenge. Whatever time and focus you invest, you'll reap the rewards in improved health—right down to your cells.

Rethinking the Medical Model: Three Pillars of Medical Care

Eric Dishman is working at the cutting edge of technology and innovation to reform our medical system. The three pillars of care that he has identified—accessibility, collaboration, and personalization—each empower us to take charge of our health.

Like Dr. Su, Eric Dishman's lifework was inspired by his personal medical odyssey. In college, he experienced bouts of dizziness and was diagnosed with a life-threatening kidney condition. As he tells it in his powerful 2013 TED Talk, his doctors told him that he had two to three years to live. Fortunately, he became friends with another patient who pointed out that his dire prognosis was based on the health outcomes of people typically in their 70s and 80s. She said to him, "They don't know anything about you. Wake up. Take control of your health and get on with your life."

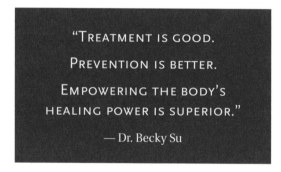

"TREATMENT IS GOOD.
PREVENTION IS BETTER.
EMPOWERING THE BODY'S
HEALING POWER IS SUPERIOR."

— Dr. Becky Su

Fighting for his life as a young adult, he came face-to-face with a flawed system that relied on specialists delivering disjointed care to "parts of us," not "all of us." Eric Dishman survived, and over the years his his treatments continue to evolve. He also became a researcher and medical policy expert who dedicated his life to "making health care a team sport." His talk, "Health care should be a team sport," can be viewed at TED.com.

If we don't "wake up" and we don't "take control of our health," bad things can, and do, happen.

My friend Susan's husband, Marco, 57, had never been ill, was a lifelong gym rat like me, controlled his cholesterol to protect himself from a family history of diabetes, and took only one medication: a statin for blood pressure. One year, over a period of weeks, he started to experience increasing fatigue and shortness of breath. Like a lot of guys, and women too, he didn't tell his partner the details of what was going on. Then one weekend, he and his wife went for an afternoon run together. Marco could only go a few yards without slowing down to catch his breath. Of course Susan was alarmed and insisted that he go to the doctor immediately.

So far, so good. Marco went to his primary care physician the following afternoon, and she made sure that he had an appointment with a heart doctor the next day. Susan went with him to the appointment with the specialist. Various possible causes of Marco's symptoms were discussed, tests were done in the office, and other tests were ordered. Heart disease seemed unlikely but they hoped the tests would show what was wrong. That's when things went awry.

His blood had to be redrawn for one of the tests and Marco went by himself. When he left the office, he wasn't sure what the next step would be. He was just relieved that the panic seemed to have passed.

Unfortunately, both his primary care physician and the cardiologist missed reviewing the results of the redone test due to a communication snafu with the lab. Not until a few weeks later, when Susan insisted that Marco call to find out what was happening, did the cardiologist look at the results. The results were extremely worrisome. Marco was immediately sent for a follow-up scan at a hospital clinic, which revealed blood clots in both lungs. He was immediately rushed to the emergency room. The clots were so large that they were pressing on his heart, which caused the breathing difficulties whenever he exerted himself. Luckily, Marco got great care with a world-leading medical team. Taking aggressive blood thinners enabled Marco to avoid surgery and be sent home four days later.

Marco's experiences—the bad and good—could be anyone's. Eric Dishman is investigating ways to change the system to shift the balance. The recommendations in his TED Talk can seem futuristic, but his three underlying pillars are relevant for all of us now:

- **Accessibility, or what Dishman calls "care where and when you need it."** Accessibility means care that is convenient, reliable, and timely, including appointments with the professionals you need to see.

  Dishman argues that we have to untether clinicians and patients from the notion of traveling to hospitals and centers. This location-based care is especially designed to deal with end-stage and chronic disease. We end up sending sick people to places where they get sicker—in other words, hospitals.

  Imagine the role of decentralization combined with the embrace of new systems. This includes social networking and resources where we can learn about conditions and also learn from other patients. Decentralization is the basis for new systems, such as telemedicine and telepsychiatry. For example, with telemedicine, data are collected by a home monitor and sent directly to the physician for review and possibly treatment. Telepsychiatry involves technology-empowered therapy sessions or online support and review. Such options will continue to expand the role of care at home or settings nearby.

- **Collaboration, or what Dishman calls "care networking."**
The one-on-one doctor-patient relationship is a relic of the past, Dishman believes. "We have got to go beyond this paradigm of isolated specialists doing 'parts care' to multidisciplinary teams doing 'person care.'"

Gee, do I agree with that! As Dishman explains, "Uncoordinated care today is expensive at best and is deadly at worst. Eighty percent of medical errors are actually caused by communication and coordination problems amongst medical team members." Dishman believes that the future of health care is smart teams that include the patient.

- **Personalization, or what Dishman calls "care customization."**
We all are different and one of a kind. We have unique histories and personalities. Personalization is relevant and necessary for every aspect of our health habits and care, from the vitamins we take and medicines that work best for us, to the foods we eat and our goals for exercise. There's no perfect plan or perfect patient.

Similar to the principles of palliative care, one avenue of customization is to focus on what is most important to the patient. This requires the person to be aware and engaged so they can get the right care at the right time.

Care customization extends to the concept of personalized, precision medicine down to the molecular level. Precision medicine is "an emerging approach for disease treatment and prevention that takes into account individual variability in genes, environment, and lifestyle for each person," according to President Obama's 2015 Precision Medicine Initiative. The idea behind precision medicine is to enable doctors and researchers to more accurately predict which treatment and prevention strategies for a disease will work in which types of people. This is different from a one-size-fits-all approach, where treatment and prevention strategies are developed for an average person, with less consideration for the differences between individual people.

So it is becoming possible to predict what diseases for which individuals are at risk, which treatments will work best for them, and which treatments may be ineffective or even dangerous. In our lifetimes, gene sequencing and other novel ways of analyzing our health will become commonplace, including a patient's genes, environment, and lifestyle.

The Food and Drug Administration (FDA) has posted on its website information on more than 150 medications whose optimal doses can be determined by DNA screening or that should be avoided to prevent adverse reactions. For example, some specific gene variations can help identify which people are likely to respond (or not respond) to specific antidepressants. Likewise, if a woman knows that she has the BRCA gene, she can decide what steps she might take to decrease her risks of developing ovarian or breast cancer.

The latest findings about self-testing through companies—such as FDA-approved 23andMe (named for the 23 pairs of chromosomes in normal human cells)—are exciting. The worry that the information might be overwhelming for individuals and their doctors to deal with isn't turning out to be the case. People are largely happy with the knowledge they gain, though we have to remember that our genetics can provide a map of where we might end up, but our habits may take us on a different, better journey.

Don't Let the Mirror Fool You

There's an important warning about taking charge of our health. We need to get beyond how we look in the mirror and instead focus on how we feel and what our health risks are.

Although our ideal body weight has been a go-to marker of health, how we look doesn't tell us how healthy we are. According to the results of a 2017 obesity and chronic illness study by Kaiser Permanente Center for Health Research of the 1.3 million people studied, 14% of people had normal blood pressure, blood sugar, and cholesterol levels. However, the lead author states that just because they currently don't have risk factors doesn't mean that they are not going to develop them.

- 30% of obese people have normal cholesterol, blood pressure, and blood sugar levels and a 70% risk of developing a major illness.
- 50% of overweight people have normal levels of these parameters and a 50% risk of developing a major illness.
- 75% of people of normal weight have normal levels of these parameters and a lower, but important, 25% risk.

We need to know our numbers and take charge of our health. That's what my friend Bob McCleskey found out. He's the kind of guy who should be on the cover of *Men's Health.* He's ruggedly handsome, athletic, 6' 4", 190 pounds, super successful, articulate, and an all-around good person. This guy seems to have everything.

When Bob was in his early 50s, he was playing basketball, and after he came out of the game for a few seconds, he had a cardiac arrest on the bench. Luckily, there was an automated external defibrillator (AED) nearby. Even more fortuitously, one of the athletic trainers in the gym was trained on how to use it. The paddles were set in place and Bob was shocked back to life. The medics arrived quickly and got Bob to the hospital, where he received the emergency treatment that he needed to survive. Twelve months later, Bob had to return to the hospital for open-heart surgery.

It was a terrible time. Fortunately, Bob got back to good health. His physical fitness surely helped his recovery, but it masked his underlying risk. It wasn't something he could see on the outside. He was caught in what I think of as the 'mirror syndrome:' "I look good, I look fit, so I must be healthy and doing well."

Bob had had regular checkups, there was an important baseline test that he hadn't had. It was the computed tomography (CT) calcium scan, a simple test that measures calcium deposits in the coronary arteries and indicates signs of heart disease. If he'd had a scan, he would have been treated long before he faced a life-and-death emergency.

Once Bob recovered, he became a major advocate for CT scans and a supporter of the American Heart Association. Because of his activism, the number of people getting CT scans increased at the local hospital significantly, and the technicians started asking their patients if one of Bob's e-mails or talks had gotten them into the office for the test. For several months the volume of scans doubled.

The Proactive Patient: The Ingredients to Take Charge of Your Health Care

Here are specific, proactive guidelines for preventive care at midlife and getting the best treatment possible when you or a loved one runs into bad luck. When those situations arise—as they did for Marco and Bob—keep in mind Dishman's three pillars of accessibility, collaboration, and personalization and his philosophy that the best health care is a team sport.

You may think that you know all this, but you may be surprised at the nuggets that could save your life and vastly increase your chances for the healthiest, longest life possible.

Know and understand your numbers. We hear the noise of "do this, do that," and we don't tune into our bodies. We don't understand what the tests are, what the results mean, and what we're aiming for. Engage in your own health, because no one else can "make you healthy." This doesn't mean becoming obsessive or doing without pleasure and fun. It means caring about yourself. Pause there. *It means caring about yourself!*

A QUICK INTRODUCTION TO BASELINE TESTS AND NUMBERS

Discuss these with your doctor, who can help you personalize the list of tests you should take and the numbers you should try to maintain.

Body mass index (BMI)—*Desirable range: between 18.5 and 25 kg/m².* BMI is a person's weight in kilograms (kg) divided by his or her height in meters squared. Your BMI is a tool for measuring whether you are underweight, normal weight, overweight, or obese. The higher your number above normal, the greater your risk for heart disease. Many websites have BMI calculators.

Blood pressure—*Desirable range: systolic 120 mm Hg (or less) and diastolic 80 mm Hg (or less)—written as 120/80 mm Hg; the numbers can be different for people over 65.* The first number is systolic pressure, which is the highest pressure that occurs when your heart muscles contract. The second number is diastolic pressure, which is the lowest pressure that occurs when your heart relaxes between beats. High blood pressure, also called hypertension, is a major risk factor for developing cardiovascular diseases such as stroke and heart failure. You can easily purchase your own automated blood pressure cuff for convenience.

Cardiac stress test—This test often is used to rule out heart disease or dysfunction when you have a strong family history, major symptoms, or risk factors. However, be careful about having a stress test during the heat of summer. Heat elevates your heart rate and may affect your test results.

Computed tomography (CT) calcium scan—*Scores have a wide continuum. A higher score may suggest the need for further evaluation.* Some doctors say that up to 50% of people who suffer fatal heart attacks didn't know they had risk factors. The Society for Heart Attack Prevention and Eradication advises all asymptomatic men 45 to 75 and women 55 to 75 (unless they have extremely low risk) to have CT calcium scans to measure plaque and hidden coronary artery disease. (The cost is between $100 to $400 if it isn't covered by insurance.) Results should be viewed in light of any family history of heart disease or other risk factors.

Prostate specific antigen (PSA) test—Prostate cancer is second only to lung cancer as the leading cause of cancer deaths for men in the United States. Early detection is important and the PSA test can help detect prostate cancer early, when it's most treatable. This simple blood test can detect high levels of PSA that may indicate prostate cancer, but other conditions can contribute to high PSA levels. The Mayo Clinic suggests the PSA test for men between the ages of 50 and 70 and men who have an increased risk of prostate cancer. Indicating a specific PSA level as low, normal, or high is complicated because the level can rise and fall based on other conditions or medications that you may be taking. However, if you have a relative who developed prostate cancer early in life, such as in their 40s, as happened in my family, you should begin testing at age 40 so that you may have the best chance of catching and treating the cancer early.

Complete blood count (CBC)—This simple test measures the levels of your red cells, white cells, and platelets. Abnormal levels may be indicators of many illnesses.

Vitamin D—*Levels of 20 to 50 nanograms per milliliter (ng/mL) is considered healthy for most people.* It is very important to check vitamin D levels, especially with the widespread use of sunblock. Vitamin D deficiency has been linked to numerous problems, including depression and bone loss.

Cholesterol profile—*Desirable levels of cholesterol are total cholesterol under 200 milligrams per deciliter (mg/dL); LDL cholesterol under 100 mg/dL (under 80 mg/dL is even better); HDL ("good" cholesterol) higher than 60 mg/dL; and ratio of total cholesterol to HDL lower than 4.* A lipid profile has several components: total cholesterol; LDL (low-density lipoprotein) cholesterol; HDL (high-density lipoprotein) cholesterol—sometimes called the "good" cholesterol; and triglyceride levels (a type of fat that the body uses to store and transfer energy). Often, early abnormalities don't cause symptoms, so you need a blood test to know where you stand. You should be tested more frequently as you age or if you have any of the following risk factors: you are a smoker, are overweight or obese, have diabetes or high blood pressure, have a personal history of heart disease or blocked arteries, or have a family history of heart attack (male relative with heart attack before age 50 or female relative before age 60).

Fasting blood sugar (glucose)—*Desired range: 70 to 95 mg/dL. A fasting glucose level above 95 mg/dL is considered prediabetes.* High blood sugar is a signal of prediabetes and diabetes. You can buy a home-use glucometer at a drugstore for less than $25.

A1c—*Desirable range for people without diabetes: between 4% and 5.6%.* The A1c hemoglobin is a measure of the average blood sugar range over an individual's previous three months. It's also known as *glycated hemoglobin* and gives a more accurate view of someone's risk for diabetes or adequacy of diabetes control. Values between 5.7% and 6.0% indicate prediabetes. Over 6.0% is considered diabetic territory.

Know your family history and propensity for disease. Two truths stand alongside each other: you need to know your family history when it comes to health, and you need to know that your family history isn't your destiny. Talk to your siblings and your parents, aunts, and uncles. Look at photo albums to gain insights into your ancestors' health and retrace your family tree. You might have good family history, with family members who have lived healthily and dementia free into old age, or you might have a family history of diabetes or heart disease. Remember, the choices you make can change your family history, starting with you. You can change your genes and extend the life of your cells (as we'll learn about in the next chapter), and you can have more vibrancy, optimism, and purpose that make life joyful and meaningful.

Know the limitations of doctors and other health professionals. It's scary to realize that even doctors and medical professionals know how flawed the medical system has become. When it works well, modern medicine is truly a miracle. The promise of greater accessibility, collaboration, and personalization offers hope for better health as you get older.

Make sure your care is customized to you and your needs. Your health care should fit your specific condition, lifestyle, and priorities. (For example, you may have to consider costs, depending on your insurance coverage). There are no one-size-fits-all approaches anymore. You want to choose approaches and treatments that are as targeted and specific as possible.

Become knowledgeable about your health habits and health risks. For better health outcomes, become more knowledgeable about your body, your health issues, the conditions you're dealing with, and the underlying science of health and your conditions, which we'll explore in the next chapter. You will feel, and be, more empowered.

Take the Time to Find the Right Doctors and Question the System

I can't emphasize it enough: too many of us spend more time evaluating a new car that we're going to own for four years than we do the person who might help keep our hearts working properly. Here are some suggestions for choosing health professionals:

1. **Insurance:** Check whether the doctor you want to see takes your insurance and is accepting new patients.

2. **Location:** Look for health care practitioners in your geographic area. You don't want to avoid seeing the doctor just because the office or clinic is inconveniently far away. At the same time, you don't want to choose a doctor just because the office is a few minutes closer. If you were going out for dinner, you would travel to the best restaurant for your taste and style. Be willing to travel to access the best doctors.

3. **Recommendations:** Get recommendations. You can ask family, friends, colleagues, or other doctors whom you trust. You can look at reviews on various sites. Get a sense of the doctor's thoroughness, communication style, after-hours and on-call practices, and overall office management. Then make sure you check on training, board certification for specialty and hospital affiliation, and your state's medical board of licensing for any complaints or disputes.

4. **Introduction:** Ask for an introductory visit (15-20 minutes).

5. **Staff:** Evaluate the support staff you see in the office. Are there nurses, medical assistants, and medical technicians present? Do they seem happy? Did you have positive experiences with them?

6. **Action:** If you're not happy with the care you're getting, take action to get a new doctor, especially if you've already expressed your concerns to your doctor.

A FEW ADDITIONAL NOTES

- If you're too sick to go to the doctor during office hours, call your doctor and speak to the on-call doctor or nurse. If your problem doesn't seem serious (such as a sore throat that might be a strep infection, or an eye infection before a holiday weekend), you can consider an urgent care clinic near you. **In case of a medical emergency, you must go to the emergency room or call an ambulance or 911.**

- Use similar methods to identify alternative and supplemental health services, such as nutritional counseling or physical therapy.

- Consider finding a doctor trained in integrative medicine (combining Eastern and Western and other approaches) or a specialist who is board certified in functional medicine (a medical approach that focuses on your whole being, including how your life is going, your laboratory tests, and any underlying imbalances in your body.

When You're a Patient: Basic Guidelines

Here are a few guidelines for taking control of your medical care.

- **Keep a daily health journal and bring it with you to doctor appointments.** Remember, you know your body best, and a health journal or log is a powerful tool for you to accurately communicate your health status to your doctor. I've been keeping one for years. I note my sleep, weight, blood pressure, and blood sugar levels (because I'm at risk for developing diabetes) every day. Most days, I'll record the number of steps I took or the amount and type of exercise I did. If there are changes in my baseline health, I'll note those, whether that's fatigue, pain, cravings, or anything else. This might not feel natural to you, but don't blow off this recommendation. Investing this small amount of time to document your health numbers—and how you feel—will support you as you seek a healthier, longer life span.

- **If you have a medical issue that is not resolved, clarify the next steps and bring a health advocate with you.** You need to be absolutely clear when and how you, as a patient, will get follow-up. If you're in the middle of stressful treatment—and all treatment is stressful—make sure you bring someone with you, whether it's a spouse, trusted friend, or relative. They will ask the questions that you are too distracted to focus on. They will help ensure that you know exactly what the next steps are. Are you waiting for test results, coming in for a follow-up visit, seeing a specialist, or getting a second opinion?

  My wife, T, was a practicing senior nurse for many years. Now she volunteers to help people through the challenges of major medical issues, making sure that care is coordinated, the right procedures are being done, and alternatives are being considered. She knows the language and emotional intelligence within the medical culture, and she can tell if a practitioner is truly busy or just lazy. She can challenge practitioners and hold them accountable for what's in the best interest of the patient. Medical advocacy like this is a growing professional field, and there are several national organizations of professional health advocates that you can use as a starting point. You might also ask for recommendations from the social workers at your hospital. I especially recommend that you have a social worker when you have a prolonged illness or major surgery pending.

Any medically licensed person can be a health advocate. Depending on the complexity of your condition, and your familiarity with medical decisions, you might look into having one. They cost about $60 to $120 an hour, depending on where you live, and there are doctors and nurses in most areas who do this.

Years ago I had surgery, and a day or so after the operation, I was taken down to the radiology department so the doctors could monitor my progress. I was parked on a gurney and left there, in the cold basement of the hospital, for an hour. I was unable to walk to go find help. I could see nurses behind the door of the break room nearby, but they couldn't see me. I was yelling and yelling for help and finally, a nurse came out and asked me if someone was coming to get me. I said, "That's a great question!" After all that, someone eventually went to get me help so I could get the X-ray done. This story is a prime example of what can happen if you don't have a health advocate with you before and after surgery.

- **Seek the highest level of care appropriate to the conditions you are concerned about.** Ideally, your care is personalized for your age (for example, try to work with a geriatrician if you're over 65) and to receive care from the most highly trained doctor that is available to you. Although you do not need to consult a specialist for every condition, be sure that the person you see has the background and training necessary to perceive when something is out of balance.

  A note about cancer diagnosis: If you've been diagnosed with cancer, especially a rare one, don't leave your care up to just any oncologist. There is a service called *Cancer Treatment Navigator* (cancertreatmentnavigator.com) that helps you find top oncologists for your specific type of cancer. Medicine is highly specialized, and this is just one example of efforts you can make to find the best care possible, no matter what illness you face.

- **Be aware that training among health professionals varies dramatically.** When you choose a primary care physician, select someone you believe keeps current and who has the interest and training to understand the nuances of health care. Are they always talking about their golf game or the stock market? Do they get carried away discussing their personal issues, or are they focused on your concerns? Are they easily able to cite medical literature and their past experiences with particular conditions or diseases when talking about your health?

There is a reason physicians who provide primary care and specialty services receive seven to ten years of training beyond their college years to evaluate and manage medical issues. Make sure that your provider is board certified in his or her specialty, be it family practice, internal medicine, or gynecology. Look for referrals from other physicians, and check out reviews and licensure.

- **If you think that you need a screening test, whether or not you are at high risk for a condition or disease, the burden of proof as to why you don't need it is on the provider.** Your doctor might believe that some tests you request are unwarranted. Ask to see the literature on which the doctor is basing his or her recommendations. This also brings up the issue of misaligned incentives. The physicians may not want to offer a test because they feel it is not cost-effective or that a less expensive alternative might be appropriate. Depending on the response, you can offer to pay out of pocket, consider using affordable home versions of the tests, or seek help elsewhere.

- **Denial is a powerful mechanism.** When it comes to your health concerns, be honest with significant others—even a close friend—and let them know about pending medical issues so they can help you remain in charge of your health.

- **Be assertive, and make sure that you get answers to your questions and feel respected.** Even doctors need to be assertive when it comes to their own care. You don't want to become overwhelmed with information, but each person needs a different amount of explanation and repetition. You want to get the information you need in a form you can understand.

- **Hold your physicians accountable.** Many people fear that if they get assertive, their doctors won't like them and won't do a good job. They want to think of their physician as their friend. Your physician can be approachable and caring, but that's not the same as being your friends on social media or anywhere else. It clouds objectivity and responsiveness.

- **No news is not necessarily good news. Make sure you see copies of your test results.** Tests get misfiled, lost, or forgotten. If someone ordered it, you need to see it and understand the results. Even routine labs, including blood work, should be reviewed carefully. You should be notified of what they show, what's normal, what's low, what's elevated, and what needs to happen in response. If you go to another location for tests, such as for breast cancer and bone density screenings, you need to get those results and have them explained to you. It's a good practice to keep all your records in one place at home. Test results can be wrong.

On one occasion I had a calcium scan and it was 10 times higher than my previous scan result. I knew I wasn't eating that much bacon. I was freaking out. What could be going on? I couldn't have another scan to double-check because it was too much radiation for my body. So I decided to go to a doctor who runs medical tests for astronauts to get his opinion about my results. The first thing he said was, "These scans are horrible. There's something wrong with the machine that did these." He called the hospital that did the scans and found out that the scanning machine was five years past due for a software update—way overdue—so the test was wrong. I was fine. It was the machine that was sick. This gets back to the idea of questioning the system and knowing your own body really well.

- **Understand the medical records and communication system used by your doctors and care providers.** There typically is a lack of continuity in health records across many settings. Some health records are written and others are electronic. Doctors are now using electronic prompts to follow up on results, but those technology solutions are not infallible. Sometimes physicians feel uncomfortable sending digital information due to privacy concerns and have firm rules about sharing information with other health care providers. Consent restrictions sometimes get in the way. If you have copies of your records, you can control them the way you want to.

- **Learn how to have the best communication possible with your doctor.** Ask if their office is using an electronic system, perhaps with e-mail or texting features, and how to best follow up with the office, nurse practitioner (if there is one), and your doctor. Find out what to do in an emergency, too. Some doctors give out their cell phone numbers, and others will have one of their partners on call if they are unavailable.

- **Get a second opinion, particularly if your life is at risk.** Always seek a second opinion if you are uncomfortable about a diagnosis or treatment or when there are significant choices to be made about the best treatment options. Never let someone take away your hope without a fight.

When we don't add to our wellness with healthy habits, we're actually wearing down our bodies. Remember, there is no stasis. We're either strengthening our health or weakening it, as you'll see in the rest of the book.

Your Healthy Edge

DEVELOPING WELLNESS

Understanding your own body is paramount to having good health and creating longevity. Here are a few ideas to help you become a *you* expert and be the one in charge of your health and health care.

- ☐ Keep a daily journal to track your weight, blood pressure, blood sugar, steps taken, and sleep, and how you feel each day overall.

- ☐ Create and maintain a comprehensive list of prescriptions, supplements, and over-the-counter medications for your doctors to review when you visit them.

- ☐ Thoroughly research any medical practitioners you need to see by investigating their reputations, board certifications, and if they faced, or are facing, medical malpractice lawsuits.

- ☐ Document your family's health history.

- ☐ Visit an integrative or functional medical practitioner to better understand and heal the underlying causes of your health problems, rather than just treating the symptoms.

- ☐ Hire a medical advocate if you are facing a complex diagnosis or are having major surgery.

- ☐ Be assertive in your doctor appointments to make sure that you get all the information you need, presented in an understandable and useful way.

- ☐ Consider the types of support staff (nurses, medical technicians) present to help you and the physicians. These are the people who will help you first in an emergency.

Be Continually Curious

CURIOSITY, THE SCIENCE OF AGING, AND WHAT THEY MEAN FOR OUR HEALTH

"Aging and death do seem to be what Nature has planned for us.

But what if we have other plans?"

—BERNARD STREHLER,
BIOGERONTOLOGY PIONEER

After my health scare, I became very curious about the science behind health, illness, and longevity. I think if you follow your own curiosity about life and health, it can really help you live a longer, healthier life. In this chapter I explain:

- Your body is designed to keep you well, not sick, and the programming of your cells' life spans is not fixed.

- After age 30, your body's functional reserve begins to dwindle and hits an aging cliff. It happens again at 45 or 50. This is why you have to take more care to maintain your health as you age.

- Telomeres protect cellular health. If you in turn protect your telomeres through healthy habits, you can expect to have a longer life span.

- Epigenetics is an environmental stamp that can be passed on genetically. If the environment and/or behaviors are changed, epigenetics can mitigate genetic predispositions to disease.

- Currently, there is more promise than substance to any pill that says it can reverse aging.

- Learning about health and health care is worth your time. Monitor trustworthy sources or attend lectures to feed your curiosity and stay up-to-date on health topics that are important to you.

Change your mind, change your health. Being continually curious about health means taking charge of your health by taking charge of what you know: Are you willing to learn something new about the aging process instead of passively accepting the old ideas that are not supported by the latest research?

The healthiest older people I've ever met have stayed fascinated and curious about the world no matter what their hardships or health. Their curiosity and learning keeps them engaged and connected and is often part of a powerful purpose.

One of our residents at Aegis Living loves to tell stories about traveling to 150 countries. At age 97 she seems at least 20 years younger than she is. Quiet and composed, and a bit of an introvert, she's a fast and engaging talker. She went to graduate school in psychology, which seems remarkable given her age, and worked for the Red Cross during World War II. Her assignment was to travel to bases to set up social clubs for the soldiers since the military couldn't do it. The men at that time were lonely, and she was treated like a caring den mother during the time it took her to get each place up and running. Then she'd move. She did that work for 50 years in all. Once, she and her husband went around the world without a single reservation. They'd hop on trains, planes, and buses and stayed at bed-and-breakfasts, using sign language to get around. If you ask her what place she liked best, she'll tell you, "Where I'm at."

That same spirit of curiosity about your health plays a unique role in your life. Even if you're not a science type, knowledge about the biology of aging—coupled with experience—can inspire you to take action. I hope this chapter will give you an accessible introduction to the exciting science about your health potential at midlife. It's good news!

Each of the following habits highlights key scientific insights that underlie any changes we make and highlights strategies that can make the difference in your well-being.

CHAPTER TWO

Aging as a Risk Factor— Not a Prescription—for Decline

In the last chapter, I made the point that aging and decline are not synonymous. Science is proving why that is true. Once thought to be inextricably connected, aging and illness are now understood to be two separate trajectories. You will grow older but your aging process may not involve illness.

The common feature for nearly every major health problem—from hypertension and diabetes to cancer and Alzheimer's disease—is that the risks increase as we get older. Why is that? What is inevitable and what is not?

> AGING AND ILLNESS WERE ONCE THOUGHT TO BE INEXTRICABLY TIED TOGETHER BUT ARE NOW UNDERSTOOD TO BE TWO SEPARATE TRAJECTORIES. YOU WILL GROW OLDER BUT YOUR AGING PROCESS MAY NOT INVOLVE ILLNESS.

There is a whole world of scientific research proving what Eastern and alternative medicine have advanced for generations. Our bodies are designed to keep us well, not sick. Even so, our biochemistry has inner mechanisms that slow down our functioning as we age. Fortunately, we have some control over how we "turn on" and "turn off" our cellular health. Thus, our rate of aging is determined by a combination of our genes, lifestyle, exposure to harmful chemicals and diseases, access to health care, physical activity, and the foods we eat.

While the majority of our bodily functions peak shortly before age 30, most of them remain adequate because most organs start with considerably more useful capacity than the body needs. This phenomenon, called functional reserve, is what allowed me to get from my 30s to my 50s still in one piece, despite pushing my body. We have a lot of built-in redundancy we can draw on to recover and recharge.

Marco's story is another example: Although his heart function was reduced because of the pressure from the blood clots in his lungs, he had enough surplus function to literally protect his life. As one doctor explained to me, "It's actually quite hard to die. We're designed with multiple, duplicate, oversourced supplies of cells, blood vessels, nerves, and even lungs."

Grapes to Raisins:
Signs of Our Programmed Aging

Our natural process of maturing and aging begins at the moment of conception. Think of a baby as a perfect grape: delicious, plump, and full of juice. Over time, that baby grows into an adult and physically peaks at the ripe young age of 30. Up to that point, our bodies have produced more cells than we need and have repaired themselves rapidly.

Once we pass age 30—our first aging cliff—we have to take more care to maintain our overall health. At 45 or 50 we reach a second aging cliff as the pace of cellular decline accelerates. Eventually, our once plump and flexible bodies become tighter and stiffer and then become dried out and wrinkled, like a raisin. Gradually at first, and then more noticeably, our eyes, our skin, and the cushions between our joints dry out. We harden, like those imaginary raisins, and we lose strength as our muscle is replaced with fat.

None of us can ignore the outward signs of aging—the gray hair, the drooping body parts, vision that seems to get worse by the week, and that near-universal complaint of disappearing waistlines and expanding abdomens. In fact, by the time we are age 75, our percentage of body fat, and its greater distribution in our torso, typically doubles from what it was during young adulthood. We've all had that startling midlife moment when we look in the mirror and don't recognize ourselves.

It's always struck me that when we're plump and juicy newborns and toddlers, there are few differences in overall health and vitality among children of similar ages. However, by the time those same children reach the age of 50, their physical differences are obvious. Some appear younger than their biological age and some appear older. Some are mostly healthy and others are not.

The Life and Death—and Aging—of Our Cells

The aging process all starts—and ends—with our cells. We are either helping or harming them with our habits of health, just like Dr. Su's sandpile metaphor.

Our trillions of cells are organized into different tissues and organs. Many of these cells reproduce continuously. Others proliferate on demand, such as white blood cells, which multiply in response to an injury or to fight infection.

Other types of cells do not typically regenerate, such as those in the heart, muscles, and nerves—they live for decades. As time passes, those cells die, outpacing the production of new cells, leaving us with fewer cells and less capacity to repair the damage that occurs in our bodies. Some of our organs become damaged, and we may develop health problems that we could have resisted when we were younger.

Here's what most of us don't know or understand: the programming of our cells' life spans is *not* fixed. Essentially, you have a lot of control over the life expectancy of your cells. This is a really big deal when you think about it. We are not at the mercy of chance or heritage.

In 1965, a biologist named Leonard Hayflick, PhD, noticed that individual cells grown in cultures reproduce by dividing and replicate copies of themselves a finite number of times before the division process stops. They live for a while after they stop dividing during a period called senescence. Once a cell reaches the end of its life span, it undergoes a programmed cellular death called apoptosis. Hayflick discovered that the cells would only divide between 40 and 60 times, known as the Hayflick limit.

There are multiple reasons why a cell should be programmed to die after a certain point. For example, during development of human embryos, cells that were needed in the first days and weeks of growth are not needed at later stages, say when tissues need to be remodeled into fingers and toes.

> HERE'S WHAT MOST OF US DON'T KNOW OR UNDERSTAND: THE PROGRAMMING OF OUR CELL'S LIFE SPANS IS **NOT** FIXED. ESSENTIALLY YOU HAVE A LOT OF CONTROL OVER THE LIFE EXPECTANCY OF YOUR CELLS.

Programmed cellular death can benefit us when cells have damaged genes, which may hasten aging and age-related diseases. It can also defend against the growth of cancers. Even though cancerous cells may experience uncontrolled growth, they still have a defined life span and will eventually die. Chemotherapy agents, for example, are designed to hasten this process in order to accelerate cell death in cancerous cells.

These discoveries lead to the one that's relevant for us. Geneticist Richard Cawthon, a student of Hayflick's, found that when he removed the nucleus of an old cell and replaced it with the nucleus of a brand-new cell, the old cell acted like a new cell. The formerly old cell divided rapidly, as it did earlier in its lifetime, eventually slowing its cellular division as it aged, before stopping altogether at senescence. The key to the Hayflick limit was found in the cell's nucleus where its DNA is housed. It is this genetic material that determines the cell's individual life span.

Telomere Protection

So stick with me a little bit more. The ideas in this chapter are about stretching our minds—curiosity is good for the mind and body—and expanding our understanding.

Before Hayflick's discoveries, cells were thought to be capable of immortality. This new information suggested that our life spans were preordained. Our cells would divide and reproduce a set number of times and that would be that. We would live as long as our cells lived—and then sputter to a halting stop at the appointed hour, if we hadn't succumbed to illness or accident already.

Then in 1978, a bit more than a decade after Hayflick's original work, the discovery of telomeres reignited the theory of cell immortality, or life extension.

To refresh your memory of high school biology, DNA is the fundamental unit of our genetic material and it's composed of sequences of subunits, our genes. These are arranged along twisted, double-stranded structures, called chromosomes, in the nucleus of our cells. At the ends of the chromosomes are telomeres. These are repetitive strings of DNA found at the ends of the chromosome. They act like protective sheaths. Like the plastic ends of shoelaces, they keep the DNA laces from fraying. However, the telomeres at both ends of each chromosome aren't indestructible. They shorten with each cellular division.

Eventually, after many divisions, the telomere is depleted, and apoptosis, or cell death, begins. Shorter telomeres are associated with shorter life spans. They may indicate older or damaged cells related to increased inflammation and weakened immune systems. Studies have revealed that people over 60 with shorter telomeres had triple the risk of dying from heart disease, were eight times more likely to die from infectious disease, and were at greater risk for cancer.

If you want to get your telomere lengths tested, there are several services available. Life Length, TeloYears and SpectraCell are popular ones, and the testing process generally works like this:

1. You give them your contact information and payment and answer to a few questions online.

2. One of their authorized physicians will review your information and then authorize the telomere length test.

3. An at-home sample collection kit is sent to you.

4. Use the sample collection kit to get one or two drops of your blood and then send the sample in for testing.

5. Results come to you in the mail in three to four weeks.

Our everyday habits and environments are associated with reduced telomere length, including the consumption of sugary sodas, exposure to pollution, and depression. Biological researcher Elizabeth Blackburn looked at the role of stress when she studied 58 women who were caregivers for sick children and compared them to women who had healthy children. The women in the group with sick children had cells with a biologic age 10 years older than their stated age. Stress was taking a huge toll.

Blackburn made another Nobel prize-winning discovery. In 2009, Blackburn and her team at the University of California, San Francisco, discovered the enzyme telomerase. This enzyme actually adds back DNA when the telomeres are wearing down, reversing the shrinking of these protective strands.

Science is proving what our mothers told us is correct. Eating well, getting exercise, having a reasonably good attitude, and managing stress ("don't sweat the small stuff")—in other words, all the habits I talk about in this book—actually increase the production of telomerase and the length of our telomeres. Meditation does more than calm us; it helps maintain our cell health.

Mitochondria and Inflammation

While cell death is the underlying basis for the aging process, it is difficult to distinguish between the changes occurring due to the passage of time and those that occur as a result of conditions such as high blood pressure, infections, and environmental stresses. Many researchers now believe that telomere shortening is more of a *symptom* of aging than its cause.

The engines that fuel our cells, our mitochondria, convert food sources into energy. They're like mini batteries keeping our cells going. As our mitochondria age and become damaged, they produce less energy, essential to the repair of our DNA. Decaying mitochondria thus interfere with cell replication, cell health, and the process that clears the body of cells that no longer reproduce but have not yet died. It's like having your refrigerator filled with vegetables that have passed their prime but are not yet moldy, indicating you need to throw them out. They take up needed space and may cause the bad smell you can't locate.

These cells with decaying mitochondria start accumulating in your organs, leading to inflammation—and inflammation is associated with or is the cause of many of our health challenges. (I'll talk a lot more about inflammation in the Eat for Life chapter.)

Your Genetic and Epigenetic Story

So what do telomeres, telomerase, and mitochondria have to do with your everyday life?

Your cells have a natural lifecycle with two masters—your genes and your environment. It's similar to the nature-versus-nurture debate when it comes to gender differences. Some gender attributes are genetically based and appear automatically at birth (differences in genitals, for example) or due to hormonal changes at puberty (a boy's deepening voice, a girl's menstruation). Other attributes are turned on and turned off or enhanced or toned down as a result of social cues, personality, and life events (assertiveness, risk-taking, emotionality).

While your genes are powerful predictors of health, longevity, and predisposition to certain diseases, they're only part of your story. You can think of genetics as the first or second act of the five-act play of your life. They set the action in motion, and like characters that come and go at particular moments, they have specific roles that evolve over the plot of your life.

Cardiologist and holistic health leader Dr. Guarneri explains:

That's why you don't have a nose coming out of the top of your head: because the nose genes get turned on in the right place at the right time in the embryo. As people expose themselves, and their genes, to different environments, certain genes will get turned on and turned off.

Dr. Guarneri emphasizes:

The important thing is that we know that genes are just the tip of the iceberg. We see that 70% to 90% of the chronic diseases we diagnose are related to environment and lifestyle. The way I teach it to my patients is this: If you have a tree and your tree has some sick fruit on it, you can cut off the fruit or you can look at the soil and you can fix the soil. The soil is your nutrients. It's your clear air and water that's not coming out of plastic bottles that have toxins. It's fitness and sleep and the way you respond to stress and tension. It's your biofield, and all the microorganisms that live in your gut, and so on. All of these things interact with your genes to determine whether you get sick or you stay well. This is why identical twins, genetically identical at birth, can have totally different genes turned on and turned off at midlife.

Epigenetics plays an important role in your genetic expression, too. Epigenetics affects how cells read genes. It is also related to the environmental stamping that is passed on to us through our DNA. You might be very healthy and think you have great genes—and you could be right. It is also possible that your grandfather, who worked in the coal mines and luckily remained perfectly healthy, nonetheless experienced environmental damage to his DNA, leaving behind damaged cells with a propensity to develop lung cancer. Through epigenetics, this environmental stamp can be passed on genetically.

> "70% TO 90% OF THE CHRONIC DISEASES WE DIAGNOSE ARE RELATED TO ENVIRONMENT AND LIFESTYLE."
> — Dr. Mimi Guarneri

According to our new understanding of epigenetics, if your father died young from heart disease, you may have a predisposition to developing heart disease due to genetics. However, your environment and lifestyle choices will play a major role in determining whether or not this happens. Likewise, just because you don't have a genetic predisposition to developing a particular disease doesn't mean you won't develop it.

There's one more twist—pun intended—to your genetic code. Family studies suggest that the genetic component of life expectancy is especially strong in the humans who live the longest. Researchers believe that longevity is, in part, determined by "longevity assurance" genes. These variations of certain genes may increase life spans and enhance resistance to environmental stresses. According to Miook Cho and Yousin Suh of the Albert Einstein College of Medicine, people who live to 100 often display unique, healthy metabolic signatures when compared with average elderly individuals. Exceptional longevity seems to be coupled with exceptional resistance to diseases that cause earlier death. Stuart Kim from Stanford University has identified five longevity genes in the laboratory—including one that determines blood group, another involved in the immune system, and a variant linked to the development of Alzheimer's disease.

Not everyone in the family gets the same inheritance, or the same environment, as we see with our Aegis Living residents. Some of the most vibrant people in our communities had siblings who died in their 60s and 70s.

Anti-Aging "Cures"

When I started my own health journey and became maniacal with my investigation into healthy aging—and possible cures—I was hoping that a magic pill was just around the corner. I was fascinated with the subculture of life-extension searchers and researchers. However, the findings of aging science made me realize that the quick-fix "Jiffy Lube" approach would never provide the deep healing and longevity of healthy habits. Our habits have the biggest impact on the longevity of our cells, the inflammation that makes us vulnerable, and the impact of our genes on our individual health.

Eventually, there will be pills and approaches that enhance our biology.

Right now, large numbers of entrepreneurs are promoting substances touted to forestall or reverse aging. These are based on naturally occurring compounds and proteins in the human body that play a role in the aging process. There is more promise than substance to these claims at this time, but I want to discuss a few of them. Some are based on sound science and though they may not lead to the magic fountain of youth, over time they may lead to personal fountains of health.

A challenge of all these interventions though is that because aging is not considered a disease, it's unlikely the FDA could approve them. The FDA isn't in the business of approving treatments just to delay aging in healthy people. The ethical issues of testing and approving drugs for this population would be enormously complex or prohibitive, and the safety standards would have to be extremely high to meet the do-no-harm standard. Therefore, when people talk about doing trials with these substances, they talk about using them on people who are in various disease states, which complicates the process of measuring the success of the outcomes.

While much research needs to be done, and there are no miracles, here is a snapshot of some of the most discussed "potions" of anti-aging you'll see discussed in ads and articles.

NAD (nicotinamide adenine dinucleotide)

During aging, as was pointed out earlier, communication between a cell's mitochondria and their nuclei, or "control center," breaks down and the effects of aging accelerate. In animal studies, decline of the chemical NAD is believed to be responsible for this breakdown in communication.

When diabetic mice were given NMN (nicotinamide mononucleotide), a precursor to NAD, their normal blood sugar and glucose tolerance were restored. This discovery holds promise for treating diabetes in humans and research is underway. NAD treatment also produces younger mice, allowing 2-year-old mice to function as well as 6-month-old mice. Researchers are now looking at the longer-term impact of the NAD-producing compound in mice, including whether it will cause the mice to live a longer, healthier life. If the studies are successful, researchers hope to start clinical trials on humans.

I began taking NAD supplements to increase my NAD levels, and now I take them everyday. The benefits I experienced after taking them for two to three weeks were increased energy for my daily workouts and not feeling sleepy at times throughout the day.

Bottom line: There are several companies producing compounds that stimulate the production of NAD. As of now there is no proof these new compounds are beneficial, but research is ongoing.

Resveratrol

Another compound that showed potential in delaying age-related disease was resveratrol, a chemical found in red wine. It was first shown to increase life span in yeast and also mimics the effect created by calorie restriction (which we'll discuss in the next chapter).

Resveratrol is an antifungal compound found in the skins of red wine grapes. It is also thought to stimulate a sirtuin (a type of protein) called SIRT1, which appears to protect mice by enhancing the health of those on a high-fat diet.

In 2008, resveratrol was widely discussed in national media, including *60 Minutes* and a Barbara Walters special. Experts were saying resveratrol was the reason for the French paradox—referring to the ability of French people to eat fatty foods but remain healthy. Corporations jumped on the bandwagon to develop and market it.

Bottom line: Unfortunately, resveratrol trials have been unsuccessful in humans and most research has ceased.

Human Growth Hormone (HGH)

Some explanations of the aging process include changes due to declines in hormones such as HGH, testosterone, and dehydroepiandrosterone (DHEA). HGH is one that is of particular interest because its use is so widespread. Many anti-aging clinics have prescribed HGH therapy. However, the actual benefits of these treatments remain unclear, and the compound may actually be risky. On the upside, it produces an increase in muscle mass and skin elasticity. On the downside, HGH can cause other complications such as kidney problems, damage to the heart and lungs, and excess bone growth.

Bottom line: At this time, human growth hormone is not recommended as an anti-aging treatment.

Rapamycin

Another promising line of research involves the drug rapamycin, which has been found to extend the life span of yeast, nematodes, fruit flies, and mice, as well as nonhuman primates. Rapamycin, which is produced by a type of bacteria and has antifungal properties, was discovered decades ago in the soil of Easter Island but slowly found its way into medical use as an anticancer agent and immunosuppressant. People believed it worked by inhibiting a key cellular pathway that was labeled the "target of rapamycin," or TOR (mTOR in mammals).

When mTOR production is slowed, the cells begin a conservation process, cleaning house and recycling old proteins via autophagy, where the cell breaks down and destroys one of its own components (as opposed to apoptosis, which is cell death).

In 2009, in a large National Institutes of Health study, scientists started treating mice with rapamycin at 20 months—the equivalent of late middle age in mouse years. The treated males lived 9% longer and the females 14% longer. Rapamycin has also been shown to reduce age-related bone loss, chronic inflammation, reverse cardiac aging, and Alzheimer's disease in mice.

It has been determined that rapamycin is relatively safe for prolonged use in human patients at risk for specific diseases. For example, researchers are currently conducting clinical trials to test the usefulness of rapalogs (rapamycin-like compounds) in preventing the reoccurrence of cancer in renal and breast cancer patients. However, rapamycin may weaken the immune system, which may limit its use with older patients whose immune systems are often compromised.

Bottom line: Currently, rapalogs are being used in clinical trials for specific illnesses. The drug is not available outside of this research, so it can't be used with people for the purpose of delaying aging.

Metformin

Millions of diabetics take metformin, a drug that has been in use for decades. Like rapamycin, metformin has extended the life of mice, and it's possible it might do the same for people. It's the latest longevity craze with early experimenters, who say metformin gives them better skin, more vibrancy, and greater energy. It also has the benefit of stabilized blood sugar and blood pressure levels.

A large review of diabetic individuals taking metformin showed they had a 15% lower mortality rate than nondiabetic individuals being treated by the same doctors. That may be because metformin enhances cellular energy utilization and protects against DNA damage that affects mitochondrial function and chronic inflammation.

Bottom line: There is hope that metformin will prove to slow the aging process and inhibit diseases.

Ultimately, we are degenerating and regenerating all the time—it's just that degeneration catches up to us. Our plump, youthful grapelike cells gradually dry up, shorten, and deform into raisinlike cells. At the same time, bodies are designed to repair, heal, repair, and rejuvenate. With the habits of health I'm describing, we can maximize and even enhance our health and healthy life span. We can start by addressing what we eat. Rather than constantly struggling with food and experiencing the silent stress of a body out of balance, we can begin to reset and regain our health from the inside out.

Getting Curious and Being a Learner

Look for small ways to stay engaged and curious in the realm of health and science and in everything you do. The following section has a few ideas to get you started.

Find one or two trusted sources of information on health, wellness, and medicine. This type of knowledge is much less guilt inducing and overwhelming than the many magazines and blogs that plug products under the guise of offering how-to advice. When you have specific health issues, look at trusted sites like MayoClinic.org, and ask your health care providers for recommendations.

Some Healthy Advice:
Sources of Insight

There are unlimited ways to learn more about your health and the science of aging, but a few sources I recommend include:

- TED Talks at ted.com (search under "health") and tedmed.com
- The "Personal Health" and "Well" sections of nytimes.com—also found on Facebook @WellNYT
- *Scientific American* (digital subscription)

Think of yourself as an explorer. At midlife, many of us rethink the direction and purpose of our lives. I'm always telling people I meet and mentor—young and older—that they should try to worry less about that one all-consuming passion and start with getting curious. Say yes to new opportunities, have conversations with new people, or start new topics of conversation with the people you're closest to. Go someplace new and get a fresh view of your life and the lives of others. This mindset of exploration and curiosity applies to all the habits I talk about, including happiness, which has just as big an impact on the health of our cells as all the others.

Go to a lecture, sign up for a workshop, or take a class. Going "back to school" is a whole new experience at midlife. You never know where those life-changing insights and experiments are going to come from. So many learning opportunities are available in every town and they are worth trying. Check out your local Y, community center, community college, hospital lecture series, bookstore, or Meetup groups.

Share what you're learning. Educational science tells us that one of the best ways to learn is to teach. Share what you've discovered in this chapter with others. Explaining information helps us make sense of it and plants it in our memory. It also helps us find companions for our journey.

Get creative. Everyone benefits from multiple types of learning and we all have different styles of learning. Make a mood board or visual map of your ideal life at your healthy edge. I have a 5' × 7' vision board in my bathroom that includes my own purpose statement, pictures of things I want to accomplish, images about health and well-being, notes on how I want to treat people in my life … I add to it all the time. Why do I do this? The body follows what the brain tells it to do. My vision board helps me program by brain and body every day to go in a positive direction.

Your Healthy Edge

DEVELOPING YOUR CURIOSITY AND HEALTH KNOWLEDGE

Staying curious is a great way to lengthen a healthy life. So is staying curious about your health care and the aging process. Here are some ideas to help keep your curiosity piqued and your mind in tune with the latest health news.

- ☐ Read or listen to at least one trusted health news source each week (e.g., mayoclinic.org, tedmed.com, @WellNYT).

- ☐ If you have questions about your own health status or condition, consider doing online research (posted by trusted sources) to learn what the latest science says about your situation.

- ☐ Try an activity you're curious about (e.g., going ice skating, going to the opera, reading science fiction, writing a blog about your experience in being curious).

- ☐ Go to a lecture or take a class on a subject you want to know more about.

- ☐ Make a mood board that represents how you want to live your life in the healthiest way possible.

Eat for Life

USE THE RIGHT FOODS TO RESET YOUR METABOLISM, CRAVINGS, AND GUT HEALTH

---

*"If diet is wrong, medicine is of no use.
If diet is correct, medicine is of no need."*

—ANCIENT AYURVEDIC PROVERB

Learning to manage when, how, and what I eat continues to pay big dividends for my health. Inside this chapter I share the knowledge I've gained about a wide range of food-related topics including:

- How to deepen your connection to food, including the time you take to eat it, how much you eat of it, and which foods nourish your body best.

- The dangerous side of the food abundance in American culture, and what kinds of foods your body is really meant to process.

- Sugar's infiltration into our food system, how it feeds inflammatory diseases, and what you can do to stop its negative effects on your body.

- The role your gut health plays in your overall health. This includes keeping your gut microbiome healthy by avoiding toxic foods, stress, and environmental toxins that harm it.

- A list of foods that are clean, combat inflammation, and balance blood sugar levels.

- How fasting, restrictive eating, and cleanses benefit your body.

- How hydration works to heal your body and even improves memory problems.

- The benefits of supplements and vitamins, including the benefits of trying personalized vitamins.

For most of my life, I denied the health problems I was having and the impact of food on my health. How on Earth could food hurt me? I indulged with abandon, ignoring the reality of what I had become. I was a caricature of the unhealthy American with a bulging belly—plus all the health risks that go along with one. Clearly I wasn't using food to layer health into my life. What I could get away with in my 30s and 40s no longer worked in my 50s.

What had happened? My body had changed. My digestive tract, my metabolism, and my ability to absorb fat—all of it had changed. I knew alcohol was damaging, but I never knew that food could hurt you, too.

Just as startling, I began to learn that the food I was eating had changed, too. Damaged foods and toxins interacted with my changing—and aging—body chemistry. I felt as if I had been invaded by an alien species churning in my stomach. After landing in the hospital due to my digestive crisis, I knew I had to deal with not feeling right in my own skin. I had to heal at a much deeper level.

Many cultures naturally have a deep, nurturing connection to food that is literally baked—pun intended—into their way of life. I was having dinner with an Italian executive on a recent visit to Rome and he put it so well: "Italians," he said, "have this romance with food — it's an investment in quality, like a good marriage. The flavors, the people, the conversation, are the main meal, not the quantity of food, and the calories. Americans, not so much. They have a quick fling with food of low quality."

For Italians, and many other cultures, the romance with food means they eat slower, savor the meal and ambience, and give their brains a chance to signal that they are full. To emphasize just this point, in Europe, you don't see people lining up in cars at a drive-through to pick up fried fast food and eating while driving.

In fact, during one of my vacations in Italy I timed our dinners. They lasted between three and four hours. The average time was three hours and 12 minutes. When I came back to the United States I did the same thing. Dinner lasted a little over an hour with the average being one hour and 22 minutes. It speaks to the habit that Americans have of eating faster, more, and unconsciously—like a factory belt full of food going right into our mouths.

Until recently, the concept of food as central to our health has been divorced from the medical profession's understanding of wellness. For too long, few Western-trained physicians acknowledged that food was so important. No one knew about the microbiome (the world of microbes in our gut that we're dependent on), or that what you ate could affect your brain and the rest of your health. The idea of inflammation as an underlying cause of all kinds of illness was seen as a fringe idea, not mainstream medicine and biochemistry. However, that's what research-based evidence is leading us to understand.

Only recently have doctors started getting onboard. For example, sugar is being recognized as the new problem child of our health and diets. I think of sugar as the civilized crack—it hooked me. With Yale University researchers sounding the alarm—based on extensive double-blind studies—that sugar is addictive, toxic, and leads to serious problems far beyond our waistlines or diabetes, it brings the idea into the mainstream. There are 6 million to 7 million people in the United States with undiagnosed diabetes. If I were president, one of the very first things I'd do would be to start a campaign to let people know that sugar is a bigger problem than illegal drugs, and that it is cutting years off our lives.

Traditionally, our medical system trained doctors in diagnosing and treating discrete disorders with protocols and pills. There has been much less training to address underlying imbalances—and that starts with the foods we eat.

> **THERE ARE 6 MILLION TO 7 MILLION PEOPLE IN THE UNITED STATES WITH UNDIAGNOSED DIABETES.**
>
> IF I WERE PRESIDENT, ONE OF THE VERY FIRST THINGS I'D DO WOULD BE TO START A CAMPAIGN TO LET PEOPLE KNOW THAT SUGAR IS A BIGGER PROBLEM THAN ILLEGAL DRUGS AND THAT IT IS CUTTING YEARS OFF OUR LIVES.

Too many of us are having a battle with food. We need to realize that food is the life force fueling all our cells and well-being—*but only if we eat healthful food that doesn't harm more than help us*. I realized I needed to understand why and how the foods I ate were making me unwell and, conversely, how I could "eat to heal." I discovered it takes knowledge and a radical rethinking of what real nutrition is. We need to stop blaming ourselves for not "eating right" and start learning and practicing the habits of eating that can put us on the right path.

Here we go.

The Burden of Abundance

Let's start with the elephant in the room: abundance. That's the large metaphoric pachyderm, which is dangerous to our health and wellness.

The health shock of overabundance, the health-wrecking foods all around us, and the metabolism crisis are real. Gluttony, our desire for more, has outstripped our common sense about what's good for us. I've also learned overabundance has done more than make us overweight. The inflammatory response it causes is making our bodies swell from the inside out.

THE AVAILABILITY OF ANY INGREDIENT WE WANT TO EAT AT ANY TIME OF THE YEAR IS ACTUALLY KILLING US.

When I travel in Europe I always notice that protein servings are usually two or four ounces—not the giant portion sizes we have in the United States where more is seen as better. Europeans also don't have as much heart disease and they rank higher on the world health scale.

The availability of any ingredient we want to eat at any time of the year is actually killing us. To provide all those foods, the food industry has had to develop means to artificially enhance them. We were never meant to eat a 20-ounce steak, pumped up with antibiotics and hormones. We were never meant to eat strawberries that are bigger than a peach, or any giant-sized foods that were once eaten moderately, locally, and seasonally.

The food we eat may look healthy and appealing, but it's deceptive. Look around you. One big example is our bread, which isn't what we think it is. The bread our grandfathers ate was made of whole wheat, with the bran and the germ. With all that fiber, it was hard to chew and took time to digest. It wasn't a fast-food nation back then.

To make a product that was easier to digest, food manufacturers removed the bran and the germ, where all the fiber and nutrients are, and processed wheat into white flour, a form of carbohydrate that turns quickly to sugar, giving us a rush of energy but also overwhelming our system. Then they laced bread with additives to disguise the lack of flavor or change the texture and put in preservatives to give it a longer shelf life. That sort of bread should stay on the shelf and not go near your body.

CHAPTER THREE

Once, I was taking an early morning walk while on vacation in a small town in Southern France, when I stopped in a bakery to pick up bread and a few croissants. I couldn't resist biting into a *pain au chocolat* and felt I had to give my compliments to the baker. I told him I had never tasted such delicious bread and pastries back home in the States. We got to talking about the differences between bread in France and the United States.

I said that I have American friends who insist that they can eat lots of bread and bakery items while in France, but back home these treats give them gastrointestinal problems. He explained that when making bread in France, they let dough rise much more slowly, letting the yeast expand more thoroughly than is typical in our high speed US culture. He was essentially saying that the stomach is a heat source, an oven if you will. When dough that's been rushed through the baking process is put in the stomach, the dough will finish it's proofing, or swelling, inside a warm stomach, therefore causing all kinds of stomach ailments. I don't know if the science is right, but it makes sense to me that French bread can be easier to digest because it's not fermenting in the gut.

What this baker was talking about reminded me of experiences when I was working for the prison system. Pruno, or jail wine, was something the prisoners made. They'd get their hands on a balloon and put sugar, fruit, and water in it. The contents would make the balloon swell as it fermented, getting bigger and bigger every week. So think of your warm stomach as a balloon: the more sugar and bread (yeast) you put in it, the more the balloon swells.

I later learned that the gluten content of French wheat averages as little as 8% to 9% while American flours are often in the 15% to 16% range. The slower, more leisurely, and social way of eating in France helps with digestion, too. Our conversation reminded me that it's important to think about the quality of the food we eat and how we feel when we eat it.

Portion sizes matter, too. I enjoyed the bread, but I wasn't quickly eating an entire basketful of it. Typically, we're not only eating carbohydrates that break down faster but also eating many more carbohydrates than we were designed to. When we were evolving as humans and prehumans, the food available to us was primarily protein and fat. We hunted and fished. Carbohydrate-rich foods were only eaten when found, usually seasonally. We hadn't cultivated grains yet, so we only ate them when we came across them in the wild.

If you think of the northern climates of Europe, there might have been natural orchards that would have had very bitter fruits, like apples or cherries, which could be feasted on for very short periods of time in the summer. In the late summer or fall there may have been tubers to dig up, which would have been extremely fibrous and only eaten in limited amounts.

Scientists discovered that carbohydrates (vegetables—especially starchy ones; fruits; grains and flours; the sugars we derive from them including corn syrup, agave, and table sugar) are handled by the body differently than proteins and fats. The body is designed to break down carbohydrates very quickly. Since we're not able to use all the energy from the carbohydrates as quickly as they are broken down, the unused carbohydrates are converted into fat.

That energy storage would help plump us up for the winter months. The cold weather would come and all those "treats" would go away. Some groups might have access to fatty foods such as whale blubber or buffalo fat during the winter and could consume them for energy, along with protein, but most of their oversupply of glucose from carbohydrates would be gone. The bodies of our ancestors wouldn't have been overwhelmed with more carbohydrates than they could handle.

People's genes vary in their ability to burn fat and carbohydrates easily, which may be due to the genetic codes we inherit from our ancestors and where they evolved. For example, in a place with lots of naturally growing coconuts, bananas, or mangoes, the local people might be able to handle fructose (a type of sugar found in fruits) better than others can. However, the overabundance of carbohydrates available to us means most people in the world today are not using their fat-burning abilities in the way they were designed.

The mango diet is a perfect illustration of what can go wrong when abundance and availability leads us astray. A seemingly healthful, innocuous weight loss remedy started to take hold some years ago with its promise of eliminating unwanted fats from the body, but lots can go wrong when we assume any healthy food is healthy to eat in large amounts. Dr. Su had several patients who went to Hawaii and went crazy eating mangoes. They all came back with the same story—all sorts of mysterious rashes and other problems. It made sense because their bodies weren't adapted to that tropical ecosystem and they didn't have the capacity to break down the abundance of mangoes they consumed. More was *not* better!

All kinds of carbohydrates, particularly sugary ones and sweeteners, are available all year long, in every type of food, naturally or as an additive. Not only is sugar

SUGAR IS RUINING OUR BODIES' NATURAL ABILITY TO REGULATE OUR HUNGER SIGNALS, TAME OUR CRAVINGS, AND TELL OUR APPETITE SENSES WHEN WE'RE FULL. THE IMPACT GOES WAY BEYOND CALORIES AND INSULIN PROBLEMS (AS WITH DIABETES).

providing empty calories, it's ruining our bodies' natural ability to regulate our hunger signals, tame our cravings, and tell our appetite senses when we're full. The impact goes way beyond calories and insulin problems (as with diabetes).

Dairy, too, used to be a limited part of traditional European diets. Perhaps you would use a modest portion of pecorino or feta to flavor foods. For me, growing up in Idaho and as a young adult, I used to have dairy a couple of times a week as a special dessert, or ice cream on a weekend afternoon. When I looked at what I was really eating by the time I got to my 50s, I saw that dairy had become a daily part of my diet. I was eating gourmet cheeses, added to many dishes at home and in restaurants. Oh, and the pizza! It had more cheese than I remember from when I was a youth and had the physical reserves to digest all that mozzarella.

I've come to learn that dairy is terrible for many people, including me. Too much of it—or even small amounts if you're sensitive—can lead to massive stomach problems and inflammation.

Another "food" that is way too abundant is alcohol. At one time, in many places it was sold primarily in liquor stores or state-controlled outlets. Now it's on the shelf of practically every convenience store and supermarket. Alcohol is a legal drug that many of us abuse without giving it a thought. Often, we deny just how much we're consuming in our efforts to "take the edge off" or "have a good time."

All this abundance of carbohydrates, dairy foods, and alcohol means we're flooding our bodies with food we can't process fast enough. The effects are life-threatening.

Our Health Foundation: Understanding the Sugar Roller Coaster and Blood Sugar Balance

Julie Starkel, a leading holistically oriented registered dietitian nutritionist based in Seattle, Washington, observes food and eating like an architect who studies form, function, and place. She looks at health like you would look at building a house. If you're building a house, you start with the foundation. You want it to be level and flat, not wobbly or cracked, because it needs to support the structure being built on top of it.

With Julie's approach, managing our sugar (that includes grains and both sweet and starchy carbohydrates) and getting our blood sugar in balance is that foundation of our house of health. The walls, wiring, plumbing, and roof are our cardiovascular, respiratory, gut, and mental health—all the "healths."

Here's why this chapter is foundational. Until our blood sugar is in balance, our bodies will send all of their healing energy to try to balance it. *The body will do this at the expense of working on any other damage, illness, or other imbalances in the body.*

There's a reason for this. The glucose derived from carbohydrates is our bodies' primary fuel. Table sugar is broken down into fructose and glucose. Other carbohydrates, like grains and starchy vegetables, are broken into glucose, fiber, and other nutrients. If we don't have enough fuel in our bloodstream, our bodies will shift gears to metabolize energy from our body fat. If there's too much fuel—too much glucose—our bodies go into overload. (If the body is desperate, it can metabolize energy by breaking down muscle, but that's something to avoid at all costs.)

Sugar is highly damaging because it moves into our bloodstream so quickly and can easily overtax our body chemistry. As soon as sugar, or any carbohydrate, meets the saliva in our mouths, it reacts with the enzymes in our saliva, speeding up the process of breaking down into glucose and fructose. So when carbohydrates move into the digestive system, they are able to passively cross the intestinal lining into the gut. They just float across, like water through cheesecloth (alcohol does this too), which rapidly raises blood sugar levels.

Carbohydrates with more fiber (think lentils, sweet potatoes, avocados, raspberries, etc.) are digested more slowly because the enzymes in our mouth and gut don't break down fiber. Imagine a bunch of glucose molecules strung together like a necklace. This is one form of starch. Now imagine little enzymes snipping one glucose off either end of that long strand to break it down—snip, snip, snip. If the enzymes come to a fiber molecule, they cannot cut through it. Instead, they head off in another direction to get around it, slowing down the process. The higher the fiber in the carbohydrate, or food, the better—meaning the more slowly it will be broken down.

Fats and proteins, on the other hand, require what's called active transport through the digestive system, and they can act like a block to faster-acting carbohydrates and help avoid a fast rise in blood sugar. Proteins and fats don't break down fully until they reach the small intestines, where they connect with the enzymes that break them down and aid in transferring them across the intestinal lining. This means that a meal begun with a few bites of protein allows the carbs in the meal to be absorbed more slowly into the bloodstream and prevents sharp rises in glucose and insulin. Because this slower process of digestion slows down the increase in insulin, the body, especially the liver, can process the broken-down molecules without becoming overwhelmed. This is the primary reason why I first eat three to four bites of protein when I sit down for a meal or have a snack. It helps me keep my blood sugar and insulin levels in check.

When your body secretes too much insulin in response to eating too much sugar and too

> "UNTIL OUR BLOOD SUGAR IS IN BALANCE, OUR BODIES WILL SEND ALL OF THEIR HEALING ENERGY TO TRY TO BALANCE IT. THE BODY WILL DO THIS AT THE EXPENSE OF WORKING ON ANY OTHER DAMAGE, ILLNESS, OR OTHER IMBALANCES IN THE BODY."
>
> — Julie Starkel, MS, MBA, RDN, founder of Starkel Nutrition

many low-fiber carbohydrates, that natural hormone that is supposed to help you, instead behaves like an inflammatory chemical. Its job in life is to open up the cell membranes to allow the body to move the glucose—your fuel—from the bloodstream into your cells to feed them. Think of it like a pet opening a pet door on the surface of those .

To understand this inflammation, just imagine you were pouring sugar into a hot glass of water and you continued pouring, stirring, and dissolving until, eventually, it turned into syrup. If you have a lot of glucose running through your bloodstream, and a lot of insulin as a result, your blood will become thicker—like syrup. Pushing this crude analogy a bit further, we can imagine this "syrup" pushing both the glucose and insulin along the interior lining of your blood vessels. Because this blood has become thick, it's harder to push through the body and it creates microscopic injuries, or little fissures. The damage sets off an alarm so the body can respond and try to repair it.

That's what inflammation is: a response to some problem or damage in the body. Inflammation can be external—like an abscess on your skin, or internal—invisibly affecting vessels and organs throughout the body. The damage from inflammation triggers an immune response, which sends a horde of white blood cells to try to fix the problem.

The roller-coaster ride of sugar imbalance is at its peak when high levels of glucose, and the resulting rise in insulin, start to cause damage to the arteries. The damage triggers the body to respond not with white blood cells but with cholesterol to start a repair process. Unfortunately, the "repair" builds up gooey plaque on the walls of arteries, narrowing them.

High cholesterol is what we always hear about, and worry about, but high glucose seems to be the major underlying cause of it, or so a growing number of experts believe. Your challenge is to go back to having balanced blood sugar levels by getting off the roller-coaster of too many carbohydrates in your diet, which affects your body's ability to function well.

A Few Truths About Sugar Overconsumption

One definition of sugar overconsumption is this: eating sweetened or processed foods every day.

Here are some sugar facts that will wake you up to how serious and common overconsumption of sugar is:

- The proven dangers of sugar were hidden from us until an exposé was published by Stanton Glantz, a professor of medicine at the University of California, San Francisco, in the *Journal of the American Medical Association* in 2016. He revealed in vivid detail how the sugar industry did just what the tobacco industry did. It hid extensive findings that proved, as early as the 1960s, the medical dangers of added sugar for heart disease and other conditions. Watch the movie *Fed Up* and you'll see the willful part the sugar industry plays in America's sugar addiction.

- Many scientists say that the surge in autoimmune and inflammatory diseases like type 2 diabetes is related to all the sugar we are eating. Our pancreas can process 80 pounds of sugar a year before the sugar starts spilling over into our bloodstream. On average, Americans now eat 150-170 pounds of sugar a year. Think of eating a 150-pound chocolate Easter bunny! To put this number in historical perspective, in the 1900s we ate 60 pounds a year and in the 1800s we were only eating 18 pounds a year. Two hundred years ago we ate 10 pounds annually, mostly because only the wealthy could afford it. The high rates of sugar consumption began after World War II, when sugar rationing ended, and the making and marketing of sugary processed foods, soda, snacks, and sweets exploded in the 1960s.

- Sugar is a potent oxidant, which means it has the potential to damage the circulatory, or cardiovascular, system—and researchers are now linking this damage to the development of Alzheimer's and heart disease. For those who are modestly worried about sweets making them fat, concerns about corroding one's brain or heart should be vastly more motivating.

- Research is suggesting that sugar affects not only blood sugar levels but also high blood pressure—maybe to an even greater extent than salt. The correlation between sugar and blood pressure may indicate that we have been worrying about the wrong ingredient. I thought my blood pressure was making it harder to push my blood through my body, but in reality it was my blood sugar that was causing me to "inflate." When my blood sugar issues went away, so did my blood pressure problems.

- You're headed for trouble if you frequently consume sugar-sweetened beverages, fruit drinks, dairy desserts, candy, ready-to-eat cereal, grain-based desserts, yeast breads, or just about anything that's processed. Processed foods with added sugar include ketchup, marinades, salad dressings, many types of bread and frozen foods, and of course soda, fruit drinks, and even "healthy" foods like protein bars.

- You need to read labels and be alert to packaging trickery. Misleading labels make many foods seem more healthful than they are. For example, a snack food box will say it's a high-fiber treat, but it doesn't advertise how much sweetener it contains. One piece of good news: Recent FDA food labeling guidelines finally require labels to reveal exactly how much sugar is artificially added—whether it's called honey, agave, high-fructose corn syrup, evaporated cane juice, rice syrup, or Flo-Malt.

- The single most important link to obesity and diabetes is the sugary drink. This includes soda but also seemingly more healthful beverages like fancy iced teas, ginger ales, and lemonades.

- Fake sugar is dangerous, too. The sweet taste keeps our bodies primed for sugar craving. There is also research showing that artificial sweeteners such as aspartame (Equal, NutraSweet) and sucralose (Splenda) have been known to increase gut bacteria associated with type 2 diabetes and possibly cause weight gain, migraines, and gastrointestinal problems.

- Consuming too much sugar—even the naturally occurring kind found in fruit—can increase your insulin levels and lead to an inflammatory response that damages the lining of your blood vessels. The Dietary Guidelines Advisory Committee urges people to cut back sharply on sugars to no more than 10% of daily calories, which is about 12 teaspoons. Just know that a 12-ounce can of Coke has about 10 teaspoons of sugar.

In my initial days on my path to wellness, I didn't really know how to begin improving my eating habits. However, given my misery, I figured I could stick with something for 60 or 90 days. I knew I had to start with something very simple, concrete, and measurable to stay motivated.

Based on what I knew, I made a vow to swear off sugar. In 75 days I lost 23 pounds. Dropping sugar was the only thing, absolutely the only thing, I changed. I cut out sodas, desserts, sugar and sweetener additives in foods, and sugary cocktails. This alone wouldn't change my whole health picture, but it was a major start.

> IN MY INITIAL DAYS ON MY PATH TO WELLNESS, I DIDN'T REALLY KNOW HOW TO BEGIN IMPROVING MY EATING HABITS. HOWEVER, GIVEN MY MISERY, I FIGURED I COULD STICK WITH SOMETHING FOR 60 OR 90 DAYS. I KNEW I HAD TO START WITH SOMETHING VERY SIMPLE, CONCRETE, AND MEASURABLE TO STAY MOTIVATED.

You have to understand that I came out of the womb with a Jenny Craig membership card in my hand. I could never lose weight until my fasting blood glucose stabilized to under 90 mg/dL each morning, and I know I'm not alone. Until that stabilization happens, your body is going to think it is in starvation mode, and won't let go of the weight. Once your body thinks things are stable, it can relax and release the extra weight because it doesn't think it's starving anymore.

My personal experience with radically cutting back on sugar is one tiny data point added to the accumulated evidence. In a 2012 study funded by the

National Institutes of Health, Laura A. Schmidt, MD, tested the impact of reducing sugar in children by changing their lunch menus. Instead of consuming yogurt sweetened with sugar, they ate bagels. Instead of pastries, they were given baked potato chips. Instead of chicken teriyaki—which typically contains a lot of sugar—they ate turkey hot dogs or burgers. The remaining sugar in their diet came mostly from fresh fruit.

After just nine days, the changes in their body chemistry were noticeable. On average, the children's LDL cholesterol, triglycerides, and blood pressure dropped and their fasting blood sugar and insulin levels—indicators of their diabetes risk—improved significantly.

While I'm not saying the alternative diet mentioned in the study is ideal, it does indicate that small changes can have a big impact on blood sugar. The study makes another powerful point: the risks of sugar consumption are real.

Getting blood sugar balanced is not that hard. Once it's achieved, other health steps can be added for a personalized plan. I always suggest people start with a 90-day "no added sugar" plan like I did, and follow the "10 Guidelines for Healthy Eating" at the end of this chapter.

Getting to the Heart or "Gut" of Our Health

There's another big idea shaping the way people are thinking about inflammation and the blood sugar roller coaster. We know that a chorus of hormones determines our metabolism, appetites, cravings, and sense of satiety, but we're finding out that the control center doesn't rest solely in our brains. One could say that our health actually begins in our digestive tract, where 95% of the bacteria in the human body live. A body of bacteria lives in our digestive tract, creating a "gut" microbiome. It is part of the greater human microbiome that resides throughout our entire body.

If our blood sugar isn't balanced, we begin to have cellular injuries and a buildup of toxins. As we saw, inflammation can happen at any point in the body, but it needs to be understood at the cellular level.

So let's look at cells and inflammation. The body is made of up trillions of cells. Every cell has a membrane that keeps all the substances and organelles of the cell inside. That membrane is made of a double layer of fat. When a cell's fat molecules get damaged, they produce free radicals.

We call that damage of the cell membrane inflammation. A cell with a damaged membrane is not going to work properly. The body sends a different molecule to fix the damage. Looking at it simplistically, sometimes it's white blood cells (sent to fight infection or repair a wound, for example) and sometimes it's antioxidants, which can help neutralize free radicals.

Finally, I Understand
Free Radicals and Antioxidants

As we know, everything around us, from our fellow human beings to the air we breathe, is made of molecules. Every molecule is made of atoms, and every atom is made up of a nucleus and pairs of electrons. When atoms are missing an electron, or a group of atoms have an odd (unpaired) number of electrons, they're called free radicals.

The question is what causes free radicals to proliferate? As Julie Starkel explained to me, everything—from environmental pollutants, alcohol, and unhealthy fats, to smoking and even exercising—generates added free radicals. They can also be formed when oxygen interacts with certain molecules.

Once formed, these highly reactive free radicals, also called oxidized molecules, can start a chain reaction as they search for an extra electron in order to restore their stability. Their goal is to steal an electron from another molecule, and when they are successful, that molecule is then damaged and starts looking for an electron to steal and stabilize it. These unstable molecules can create a sequence of damaged cells that can't accomplish their function in the body, making us vulnerable to disease. On the positive side, they also can be beneficial in some ways—for example, when they act as messengers between cells or help white blood cells do their job to kill invading pathogens.

There is something that stabilizes free radicals, or oxidized molecules: antioxidants. Antioxidants, which are abundant in fruit and vegetables, are molecules that have an extra electron. They work as donors, going around saying, *Oh, you're broken! Have an electron.* Even though the antioxidant loses an electron in the process, it remains stable. Some antioxidants, like vitamin E, can be regenerated and regain that electron for themselves.

When we nourish our bodies with foods containing lots of antioxidants, meaning mostly vegetables and fruits, we are naturally healing our cells and body, transforming free radicals into normal molecules. When we consume too much sugar—which is an oxidant—we end up with more free radicals damaging cells. We have to have plenty of foods rich in antioxidants to balance out all that free radical activity.

All the eating guidelines at the end of the chapter form the basis of an anti-inflammatory way of eating. To start, here's a list of widely available foods that combat inflammation—and that fit the specific dietary recommendations outlined in the guidelines:

- **Olive oil**
- **Green leafy vegetables**, such as spinach, kale, and collards
- **Colorful vegetables**, like red peppers, beets, and broccoli
- **Nuts**, such as almonds and walnuts
- **Fatty fish** such as salmon, mackerel, tuna, and sardines
- **Fruits**, such as blueberries, cherries, and oranges
- **Spices**, especially garlic, ginger, turmeric, cinnamon, rosemary
- **Green tea**

The gut lining can develop inflammation for a number of reasons. One is eating foods that don't agree with your body and cause some sort of irritation. Another is the imbalance of certain bacteria, "good" or "bad," in a part of your intestines.

A bacterial population, as I mentioned earlier, resides in your digestive tract, forming your gut microbiome. You have 30-40 trillion cells in your body, but about 100 trillion little microbes in your intestines. In other words, those microbes outnumber your own cells about three to one.

You need these microbes for digestive health, immune health, increased bone density, cardiovascular health, and even for brain health and emotional well-being. The useful or "good" bacteria in your gut serve as a barrier for harmful bacteria and toxins. Gut microbes also work with your immune cells to help train them how to react to various invaders. They help digest fiber and also play a role in synthesizing vitamins B and K. They metabolize bile acids and multiple other compounds. Without your gut microbes, you wouldn't survive.

This simple understanding has been very important to me personally. I always felt something was wrong with my insides, even if I was in denial about how big the problem was. I'd have health issues that I'd address with a "protocol and pill" approach, but I wasn't giving my body enough of what it needed to truly heal.

The understanding of gut bacteria turns out to be one of the most important medical advances in decades, in large part because of the relationship between an imbalanced gut microbiome and inflammation.

If you eat an unhealthy diet, such as one drenched in sugars, this may result in a bacterial imbalance, which then leads to inflammation. The lining of your colon, where most of the bacteria in your gut live, is toward the very end of your intestines. The colon has a tough time getting nutrients because the body digests everything before any of it can get down into the colon. Healthy gut bacteria provide the sustenance the colon requires to stay healthy.

Gut inflammation causes breakdowns in the rest of the body and manifests differently for every person. These malfunctions can result in negative signals to the brain, possibly resulting in mental health issues such as anxiety or depression. A malfunction can also cause the immune system to go haywire, as with an autoimmune disease.

There are a host of maladaptive responses that researchers are now attributing to imbalances in our microbiome. There are so many possible insidious causes, including:

- Sensitivities to foods such as gluten, soy, or dairy proteins like casein or whey.

- Sensitivities to food additives, preservatives, artificial sweeteners, and even food colorings.

- Enzyme deficiencies.

- Antibiotics, which devastate our microbiomes because they lead to bacterial or fungal overgrowth, as seen with a recent study that showed that just one course of antibiotics will alter the gut flora for up to 12 months.

- Antacids and acid blockers. Dr. Mimi Guarneri, a leading cardiologist and president of the Academy of Integrative Health and Medicine, explains: "We have people on drugs like Prilosec and Nexium for years when they're not meant to be used for more than six weeks. Their whole microbiome changes. Then they can't absorb their vitamins and nutrients. We end up with leaking gut, causing a host of symptoms from arthritis to brain fog and heart disease."

I know that feeling firsthand. This is actually what happened to me when I was not eating correctly. My whole middle had expanded and was bloated and tender. My liver tissue had been mostly replaced with fat and my intestines were inflamed, which contributed to the swelling and discomfort. When our microbiome is out of balance, our gut and all the systems of our bodies suffer due to the inflammation that is created.

What we know about the gut is evolving rapidly and holds many possibilities for improving chronic illnesses, which are often influenced by dietary and environmental factors. Eat a generally healthy, blood sugar–balancing diet as outlined in the eating guidelines at the end of this chapter. Avoid using and consuming antibiotics whenever possible (including antibiotics in meat and poultry). Avoid using—especially long-term—antacids and acid blockers (cimetidine, Nexium, Prilosec). Stay away from potential irritants and toxins and any foods that cause your intestines to cramp or that leave you feeling bloated, vaguely nauseous, or otherwise not well. Do try a daily probiotic and eat more foods that contain live bacteria, such as yogurt, and fermented vegetables with live cultures (which is why they are refrigerated), such as sauerkraut and kimchi.

Remember that your gut health is intimately connected to your total well-being and essential to your overall health.

Stress, the Gut, and the Mind

We actually have several nervous systems in our body. The cerebral central nervous system, headquartered in the brain, is the one we know the most about. The second one is the enteric nervous system, which is centered in the gut. If you haven't heard of the enteric nervous system, you have probably felt it when experiencing butterflies or a sick feeling in the pit of your stomach. We also feel the enteric nervous system working when we experience an irritable stomach or a digestion issue.

Our various nervous systems communicate with each other. Thought-based and physically created stress are a bit like the chicken and the egg. It's not "all in our heads" and you're not crazy if you are sick to your stomach over something that upsets you emotionally. We're beginning to learn that our enteric, gut-centered system affects our minds.

Sometimes mental or thought-based stress can cause physical symptoms because we release stress hormones into the body. These hormones interfere with the production of enzymes in the gut and hydrochloric acid in the stomach. The result is poorly digested food. Then, because there's undigested food that passes through to our stools, bacteria, which are opportunistic, start chomping on it because they like to eat. It's the little bacteria inside, having a feast that are making the gas, not our bodies. The gas causes bloating and an uncomfortable feeling of fullness—often, high up. That causes bloating, because it's probably happening higher up in the intestines. The colon can expel gas easily, but when the gas is in the small intestines, it's uncomfortable and hard to get out.

The impact of maintaining an imbalance of bacteria in the gut microbiome can create a chain of events where the body is not absorbing nutrients, causing further harm.

The Benefits of Limits: Experimenting With the Restrictive Access and 5:2 Diets

What we eat for health is not necessarily the whole story, however. The old adage "Eat breakfast like a king, lunch like a prince, and supper like a pauper" points to the fact that the timing of when we put food in our bodies makes a big difference. The latest science is starting to show us why.

Eating late at night, particularly if the foods we are reaching for are loaded with sugar and fat, is a big problem. Our bodies are designed to get a break at night but instead start digesting the sugars and fats we just ate.

Many studies have shown that it's a good idea to restrict the time window for eating so that you have a long fasting stretch during a 24-hour cycle before you "break your fast" with breakfast. Early experiments with mice at the Salk Institute, in California, showed that those fed a high-fat diet but only allowed to eat within an eight-hour window during the day were healthier and slimmer than those given exactly the same food but allowed to eat whenever they wanted.

Neuroscientist Mark Mattson, PhD, at the National Institute on Aging has researched diet restrictions that used to seem extreme. While the practice is controversial, many studies have shown that restricting the timing and the amount of food you take in beyond recommended baselines can actually improve both your physical functioning and the ways your brain works, especially in the areas of good thinking and memory.

Dr. Mattson points to a study by Dr. Michelle Harvie at the University of Manchester that involved 107 overweight women, half with a family history of breast cancer and half without. One group ate 25% fewer calories than they needed to maintain their weight, seven days a week. The second group ate normally five days a week but on two days of the week they ate 25% fewer calories than needed for maintenance. This was a six-month study and 80% of the women in the study managed to stick with their diets. Both groups lost similar amounts of body weight, but the women on the so-called 5:2 diet, or the "fast diet," lost more belly fat and had greater improvement in their insulin sensitivity than the three-meals-a-day group.

As we've seen, blood sugar balance is a strong marker for improved health and lowered risks in a broad range of areas.

It turns out that if you eat three meals a day, every time you eat, the energy (or glycogen) stores in your liver are replenished so you never really use or burn the energy you have stored. However, if you fast 10 to 12 hours, you deplete your glycogen stores and then mobilize the fatty acids from your fat cells. These fatty acids are released into the blood and travel into the liver where they are converted into what are called ketones. Fasting for 12 hours is a great way to burn fat.

What else happens during our fast? Over six to eight hours, the liver is digesting food before turning to its other essential job: repair and detoxification. The liver digests food first because it has to get the nutrients from the food we've eaten into all the different areas of your body—that's their fuel. Only then can it draw its attention to the many processes it's responsible for when food is not present, including healing cellular inflammation and detoxifying—ridding the body of damaging or extraneous substances. Without a long enough break in the eating cycle (say 10 or ideally 12 hours), there's no way your liver can keep up with its two jobs! It neglects the second one. But with this break, your liver will have four to six hours to help boost your immunity, delay degeneration, and aid cell-level rejuvenation. When your eating habit includes limiting the period of time each day that you allow yourself to eat, you can gain a healing edge in midlife and beyond.

Restrictive eating can be taken one step further. Dr. Mattson is a leading proponent of intermittent fasting, but especially when it is coupled with exercise—a combination that seems to have a remarkable effect on the functioning of the human brain. **This effect, he believes, has its roots in ancient biology:**

It makes a lot of sense that fasting and exercise will improve cognitive function, because if you're an animal, say you're a carnivore and you haven't been able to track down prey for a couple days, your brain better be functioning well or you're not going to be able to figure out how to track down the prey. You also better be physically fit when you're expending energy to track down whatever it is you're chasing.

Dr. Mattson continues:

Cycles of exercise or fasting followed by recovery periods do two major things:

1. *Increases stress resistance and decreases the amount of damaged molecules in the cells.*

2. *Allows the cells to grow and, in the case of neurons, grow more synapses, which in the brain we think is critical for improved learning and memory. And in the case of muscle cells, they get bigger and stronger.*

Some diet and nutrition experts are concerned that low-calorie restrictions can spur cravings and binges, but the data are compelling. It's worth considering if this type of simple and concrete plan appeals to you, much like my initial sugar elimination approach worked for me.

Recently I took a big step with a 21-day cleanse. A cleanse is designed to rid your body of toxins and reset your metabolism and whole biochemistry. I eliminated all dairy, grains, and processed sugar. I lived on chicken, fish, seafood, all vegetables, and some fruit. The most difficult part was the first few days. But overall, it didn't bother me. I slept better and had more energy. Everything improved. Given the impact, I'm intending to repeat the cleanse every three months, like the way we approach our fall and spring house and yard cleanups, repairs, and improvements.

A note about fish—I gave up eating beef on a weekly basis. I now eat it about two to three times a month, and I turned to fish as a substitute, wanting a healthful protein and the omega-3s. However, I tested my mercury count, which was five times higher than it should be. My wife's was 10 times higher. Our lead counts were off the charts, too.

We had our house tested for lead and mercury, our water, our antiques, our cars … then my doctor says to me, "Why don't you give up fish for 30 days?" We did it for a month, got tested again, and the results were normal.

Even though we were eating the highest-quality fish, this story illustrates that our waters are so polluted that even fishing licenses say *don't eat fish more than two times a week.* It's a warning label on your fishing license! So every year I go off fish for a while to get the lead and mercury out of my system.

One-to-Five Eating Philosophy

The problem with diets is that we tend to eat between bookends of extremes. How many times have you known you were going to go on a diet and then ate every bad food imaginable the day before? The rational was, "I'm going to be deprived, and I'm going to inhale all these bad foods before I can't have them anymore."

Controlling our diet and weight is really about conscious eating—being truly aware of what we put in our mouths.

Even though I've lost 50 pounds, no one is going to think I'm a skinny guy. To make matters worse, because I'm writing this book, I feel scrutinized about what I put in my mouth. To maintain a healthy diet and relieve that sense of being in a fishbowl, I've found the one-to-five eating philosophy comes in handy.

If you eat like a one, the bookend on the left, you are ultra conscious about everything that goes in your mouth. No refined sugar, very few bad carbs, minimal portions, no fried food, no dairy, and maybe no meat among many other highly nutritionally conscious endeavors. Essentially, you are following a minimalist diet and eating about 800 calories a day.

Two eaters consume mostly fish and seafood. They are OK with vegetables of all kinds but no bread, very little bad starch, and no dairy, and they watch portions closely.

Three eaters would add potatoes and brown rice to how a two eats, and perhaps chicken or lean beef a couple times a week to their meal plans.

Fours build on the threes by adding bread, beef, some sugar, and maybe a processed food a couple times a week to their diet.

The bookend on the right is a five. This way of eating has no boundaries. Fives probably have chocolate milk and sugary cereal for breakfast, two cheeseburgers for lunch, fried chicken for dinner, and a big piece of cake and toffee ice cream before bed. Yes, some people eat this way.

So what's your number?

The reality of life is that it is unrealistic to eat like a one the rest of your life and unhealthy to eat like a five for any period of time. So the trick is to eat like a two to a three most days of the week, and then on the weekends you can explore eating like a four for a day or two.

Note that if you live in the four or five range, intermittent fasting can be a quick and effective weight control practice for you.

When Self-Help May Not Be Enough

If you are dealing with weight gain or other chronic issues, pain, high cholesterol, prediabetes, binge eating, or any significant concern, all the advice in this chapter is helpful, but there's no substitute for professional care, treatments (when appropriate), and lots of support. Keep these points in mind as you think about your next steps and read the next section, "Real Nutrition for a Longer Life."

- Focus on health and blood sugar balance over weight loss—even a 5% to 10% weight loss improves health and is sustainable over the long term.

- Lose weight slowly—the body fights weight loss, so be a tortoise and not a hare.

- Know that your struggles are real. Researchers are beginning to realize that obesity and its precursor—being overweight—are not one disease but many, which makes treatment difficult and results wildly variable.

- Seek the guidance of a health expert who can work with you to personalize your plan and provide the support you need. Seek out supportive people in your life, whether that's family (who are not always as supportive as we'd like with the changes we're making), a group at your local Y or church, or any other options that suit you.

- Use a health journal to log the foods you eat, along with portion sizes.

AMPK—The Longevity Enzyme: The Role of Intermittent Fasting and Exercise

Recent research is showing the powerful effect of combining extremely low-calorie diets with highly intensive exercise. The combination can have a powerful effect on the enzyme AMPK, which some people are calling the longevity enzyme.

AMPK (adenosine monophosphate-activated protein kinase), which is found in all the cells in our bodies, is now known to have a powerful role in orchestrating how we extract, store, and distribute energy from food, including how our bodies manage glucose, insulin, oxidation, and cholesterol synthesis. It may be a unifying culprit behind our health declines, which are largely controlled by our metabolic system.

Additionally, AMPK inhibits NF-κB, a molecule right in our DNA and a key overseer of inflammation, which we know is an underlying factor in all age-related diseases. When AMPK is switched on, it triggers the use of stored energy from fat, the metabolizing of fats and sugars in the blood, and the increase in production of mitochondria (again, those are our cells' batteries). AMPK also plays an important role in eradicating damaged DNA and misshapen proteins. This is important because these cells can harm the body by leading to conditions such heart disease, diabetes, and Alzheimer's disease.

Dr. Guarneri says:

If you eat a Big Mac, a bag of fries, and a big shake, the research shows that you turn on NF-κB. The minute you turn on NF-κB you start producing proinflammatory cytokines, small proteins released by cells. You end up with inflammation all over the body, a common denominator of age-related diseases. This is the exact opposite of what happens when you eat a can of sardines or a piece of wild salmon, which turn on totally different cytokines, which are anti-inflammatory.

In other words, the biggest, safest driver of plentiful AMPK is getting control of your blood sugar and your own metabolic roller coaster. The more in balance your metabolism is, the more efficient it is, the higher your AMPK will be, and the more resilient your cells.

Real Nutrition for a Longer Life

You can burn calories, but you can't burn off bad nutrition. You also can't wing your diet as you enter mid- and later life.

> YOU CAN BURN CALORIES, BUT YOU CAN'T BURN OFF BAD NUTRITION. YOU ALSO CAN'T WING YOUR DIET AS YOU ENTER MID- AND LATER LIFE.

The scientific literature and the popular media are full of experts suggesting what makes for a healthy diet and a long life. Much of their advice is sound and helpful. Find what works for you and any specific health issues you're dealing with. Avoid hype. Stick with simple approaches that fit you. Remember that all calories are not equal—500 calories of snack food and the same 500 calories of sautéed spinach have completely different effects on the growth of your cells. As my Italian dinner partner knew so well, quality matters—for your eating pleasure and your healthy life span.

Here are baseline recommendations to balance your blood sugar—the foundation of your health and your total well-being.

Water: Hydration Is Nutrition

- Water influences every process in your body. Think of it as a macronutrient that gets more important with age—the grapes-to-raisins phenomenon that becomes noticeable in midlife.

- We lose a lot of water every 24 hours, including six to eight ounces during the night. You need to replace the water you lose when you breathe, perspire, and urinate in order to maintain your blood pressure, aid your digestion, and regulate your metabolism.

- As people get older, particularly over the age of 50, they often complain of feeling tired, foggy, and draggy, not realizing that what they really are is thirsty. They may opt for a nap only to experience headaches, dizziness, dry mouth, or constipation due to dehydration they haven't addressed.

- People vary widely in their need for water, based on weight, exercise routine, body makeup, and time of year, but the traditional prescription of eight 8-ounce glasses of water a day (64 ounces daily) is a good starting place. I've found I need about 115 ounces a day. Of course if you're a petite woman you may need less. Begin the morning by drinking water and carry a refillable bottle with you throughout the day so you don't forget to drink it. Foods, especially certain fruits and vegetables, add water to your daily intake, but try to get in those eight or more glasses. We stop noticing our thirst as we get older so we must be proactive about getting the water we need. In fact, one of the first things we do at Aegis with residents who begin showing signs of dementia is to hydrate them.

- I don't know exactly when I started experimenting with hydration, but I think it was one of those "typical Dwayne" moves where I found one thing I could do without too much fuss. I could approach it like a training routine in the gym. So many reps, so many times a week. Very concrete and clear. That has always been my way to get started on something.

- I learned that alongside fatigue, gastric issues, and "foggy brain," asthma could be linked to dehydration. That sounded like me—not drinking enough water and having these symptoms. I started to drink more water every day.

- When you get up in the morning, ideally within the first 15 minutes of waking up, drink a glass of room temperature water, or even two. Drinking plenty of water upon rising is a common practice in Japan, where they have been doing it for many, many years. Why room temperature? Some believe if water is cold, it will actually inhibit your digestive tract from functioning at its best. Plus, your body has to expend energy to heat up the water to body temperature. Just leave out a bottle or pitcher of water overnight so it's ready for you in the morning. This habit lets you start your day detoxifying and cleansing your body. How often do you wake up with a foggy head and say, "Oh, I'm useless till I have my coffee"? Wrong approach. Drink water and wait 30 minutes before you have your coffee (always with breakfast or a morning snack).

- Over time, I've read up on Eastern and Western approaches to hydration and experimented to find what is right for me. Once the habit was in place, I never went back.

Alcohol

- Washington State is known for great wine and it's especially popular in Seattle to hail the benefits of a daily glass of red wine, since it's been shown in some studies to lower the risk of heart disease. But that's not the whole health story on alcohol.

- Alcohol abuse is a major reason for early death in this country. It causes everything from cirrhosis to depression to cancer to osteoporosis and is the king when it comes to killing cells. Alcohol also promotes premature aging. Falls are a significant risk in the elderly and drinking alcohol can cause them by affecting a person's balance.

- Don't fool yourself into thinking you are OK if you binge drink one day and avoid alcohol the next. A group of Harvard scientists claim that "having seven drinks on a Saturday night and then not drinking the rest of the week isn't at all the equivalent of having one drink a day. The weekly total may be the same, but the health implications aren't." There's a fine line between where alcohol actually has a positive effect and then begins to do harm.

- Among participants in their 2003 Health Professionals Follow-Up Study, modest drinkers who reported having a drink three or four times a week—a 1.5-ounce. cocktail, a small glass of wine, or a 12-ounce. glass of beer—were less likely to develop cardiac disease than nondrinkers. But while there can be some health benefits to having just one drink every day or or so (depending on your health and medication history), there are only negative health consequences to excessive drinking. In fact, most people don't realize that as we age and our bodies detoxify more slowly, the nightly beer we could handle easily at age 30 probably isn't something our bodies can process healthfully at age 60.

- The World Health Organization's International Agency for Research on Cancer classified alcohol as a Group 1 carcinogen, similar to arsenic, benzene and asbestos. The agency's evaluation states, "Alcoholic beverages at any quantity are carcinogenic to humans."

What and When to Eat

- For starters, eat real food. Given our overprocessed environment, you need to learn about what real food is and make conscious decisions about where to find it. Michael Pollan, an activist and prominent writer on the subject of food, puts it best when he says, "Eat real food, not edible food-like substances. If it doesn't look like food, don't eat it." Pollan adds additional rules of thumb that include:

  - Eat only foods that will eventually rot.

  - Eat only foods that have been cooked by humans, not machines.

  - Avoid foods you see advertised on television.

  - Remember, the produce section is where the healthiest foods are. They're the "silent foods," meaning they don't shout health claims on their packaging.

Eating Guidelines: 10 Eating Habits for Blood Sugar Balance and Anti-Inflammatory Health

There are many diets out there that are valuable. Discover which one is right for you.

Here's one very straightforward approach designed to create a foundation for your lifelong healing edge. It's adapted from the plan my nutritionist, Julie Starkel, has taught me. It's simple and has worked better than any other approach I've tried. Also, it's easy to personalize or modify for your specific health needs.

1. **Make sure you have protein as part of every meal and snack, and make your first four bites protein.** Protein is the most satiating food we eat and it takes the longest to break down during digestion, so it allows our metabolic system to function as it was designed. Our goal should be to satiate ourselves with protein and slow down and even out our blood sugar roller-coaster ride. Eating protein at every meal and snack helps us avoid rushes of glucose from sweet and starchy carbohydrates.

   Be mindful of these protein guidelines when choosing the type and amount of protein to eat:

- While many Americans get enough protein, you want to be sure you aren't one of those who don't. Very roughly, think in terms of 0.8 to 1 gram of protein per kilogram of your body weight (or your "reasonable" goal body weight). In pounds and ounces, that translates into:

> 200-pound person = 91 kilograms =
> 73-91 grams of protein = 11-14 ounces per day

> 150-pound person = 68 kilograms =
> 54-68 grams of protein = 8.5-10 ounces per day

> 120-pound person = 54 kilograms =
> 43-54 grams of protein = 6.5-8.5 ounces per day

- In terms of food and meals, a 150-pound woman might split up her daily protein intake into two ounces of protein at breakfast; one ounce of protein in a snack; three ounces of protein at lunch; another one ounce in a snack; and two to three at dinner. An ounce is about the size of an average hand's index finger. A deck of playing cards is about what three ounces look like.

- One egg generally equals one ounce. Fish, chicken, beef, and other animal proteins all vary slightly, but these estimates should be sufficient.

- You can also get your protein from legumes, quinoa, and tofu—these are common choices for vegetarians. Vegetable-based proteins have slightly lower amounts of protein so you can add an ounce or two more of vegetable-based protein to balance the protein you're getting each day. There are several reasons people choose to be vegetarian, but if you are having health issues, and you eat organic and locally raised products, it could be that you need to eat meat. Even the Dalai Lama, the leader of a religion that practices nonviolence toward humans and animals, discovered that he was healthier when he ate a little meat and stopped being a vegetarian.

2. **Eat approximately every three hours—always with protein.** If you wait too long between meals or snacks, your blood sugar will drop and that can be hard on your system. Low blood sugar has its own chemical that raises its ugly head and that's cortisol. High levels of cortisol increase inflammation by secreting inflammatory chemicals that break down muscle tissue for energy. It supports our bodies' emergency backup system for fuel. Toward that three-

hour mark, you reach your lowest blood sugar territory. You probably won't feel it right away because the symptoms come later.

The best intervention if you go too long without food is a snack of protein and vegetables with fiber—maybe a small chunk of turkey with a little cucumber, or small egg with tomatoes. That kind of snack brings your blood sugar back up so your body doesn't start producing reactive responses.

3. **Eat breakfast as soon as you can—preferably within 30 minutes of waking.** Some people take medications upon waking that require they wait 30 minutes or one hour before eating, but if that isn't the case for you, try to eat within 30 or, at the most, 45 minutes after waking up. Of course, you might be one of those people who balk at this idea, like me, thinking you can't possibly eat before 11 am. I found that eating just two or three almonds has a metabolism-raising effect similar to eating a whole meal. I also know that as we train our bodies not to be hungry in the morning, we can train our bodies to get hungry. It may also be because you ate too late the night before and have not allowed your body the 12-hour fast it needs at night.

When you eat breakfast, what you choose is very important. If you eat something that is primarily, or only, made up of carbohydrates (like all combinations of grain, sugar, and fruit), such as pastries, cereals, or even granola, you're going to drive your blood sugar up. This will cause the body to compensate by secreting excessive amounts of insulin, which is not a good way to start your day. Plus, you'll feel excessively hungry and tired later that afternoon, driving you to choose sweets as an afternoon snack as well. Instead, try eggs, turkey bacon, or even "regular" food like salad bowls with protein and vegetables for breakfast.

4. **Plan meals and snacks for blood sugar sanity.** Multiple low-glycemic snacks throughout the day may cause fewer spikes in blood glucose than the three-meal-a-day method. The timing or order can be adjusted to fit your schedule. This formula is meant to help you, not harm you with a plan you can't, or don't want to, follow. Customize it according to your needs.

Ideally, your dinner is smaller than your lunch and maybe even your breakfast. You certainly don't want a large meal after 7 pm, except on occasion. It will tax your body's whole digestive, detoxifying, and healing process.

5. **Don't count calories! Plan your plate—vegetables and the rest.** So after you have chosen some protein to put on your plate, what do the rest of your meals look like?

   Ideally, more than half your total consumption for the day is made up of colorful, nonstarchy, or low-starch vegetables. Think of dark leafy greens and cruciferous vegetables like broccoli and cauliflower. Think of red, green, and orange peppers. All the nutrients and antioxidants you need are coming from vegetables, which will go a long way to helping you not only with your cravings, weight, and gut health, but also with other health conditions that you may worry about. (You can refer to the list of anti-inflammatory foods earlier in this chapter.)

   You want to keep your total dairy to a minimum and limit your fruit to a couple of servings a day. Berries are an excellent choice because of their high fiber content.

   Julie advises her clients to "plan their plates," and not count calories or measure portions. Your plate looks about like this:

   - A third of your plate is protein.

   - Half or more of your plate is vegetables—for example, a salad and/or two vegetables.

   - For the small portion of your plate that remains—about the size of a small slice of melon—you'll eat starchy root vegetables (like sweet potatoes, parsnips, carrots, beets) or whole grains, with a preference for the root vegetable since they have more vitamins and are more filling than grain.

A Note About Gluten

The plan-your-plate approach to eating takes care of most issues with gluten. It limits the amount of grain or bread you can eat to that "slice of melon" amount. If you are sensitive to gluten, or think you are, you can eliminate it for a month and then reintroduce it in small amounts to see how you respond. If you're not particularly sensitive and you avoid processed foods with added sugars (such as sweet muffins, cake, donuts, chips, and so on), you'll avoid most of the problems that come from eating gluten—and without a lot of effort.

6. **Aim for quality.** If possible, choose organic foods and hormone-free and grass-fed meat. Wash fruits and vegetables thoroughly even if they are organic—and do it to reduce any surface soil if they are. Look for seasonal food, especially at local outdoor (spring/summer/fall) and indoor (winter) farmers markets. Though organic food is more expensive, if you avoid waste and eat smaller portions or smaller dishes when you go out, you will be way ahead in the long run—with your body and your budget. (Research shows that a family of four discards $1,500 worth of food each year; nationally, we throw away 30% to 40% of our food; and consumers waste up to 50% more food today than they did in the 1970s.)

Organic Foods: The Dirty Dozen and Clean Fifteen

While organic foods aren't necessarily nutritionally superior to their nonorganic counterparts, they are free of the toxins found in synthetic pesticides and are highly recommended. If availability or cost is an issue, you can get a list of foods that have the most and least pesticide residue, created by the Environmental Working Group. Try to buy organic varieties of the Dirty Dozen foods, or remove the skin, and eat relatively more of the nonorganic Clean Fifteen foods. Here's the 2017 list, based on the samples that were evaluated:

The Dirty Dozen		The Clean Fifteen	
Strawberries	Cherries	Sweet corn	Mangoes
Spinach	Grapes	Avocados	Eggplant
Nectarines	Celery	Pineapples	Honeydew melon
Apples	Tomatoes	Cabbage	Kiwis
Peaches	Sweet bell peppers	Onions	Cantaloupe
Pears	Potatoes	Sweet peas	Cauliflower
		Papayas	Grapefruit
		Asparagus	

7. **Aim for 12 on, 12 off— 12 hours in the day when you're not eating.** Similar to Dr. Mattson's advice, plan to eat during the hours between 6 am and 6 pm, 7 am and 7 pm, or 8 am and 8 pm. This allows your liver to do its job. The liver is critical for digestion and it takes six to eight hours for the liver to process all the food that comes in after a meal. If you eat dinner at 6 pm, your digestion process will go till midnight or 2 am. From 2 am to 6 am, your liver doesn't have to deal with food and it can attend essential repair and detox of our cells.

8. **Beware of toxins, including coffee.** Sugar can be seen as a toxin—or addictive substance—which isn't good!

   Coffee can be considered a toxin, and the FDA lists coffee as a food that contains high levels of the carcinogen acrylamide. No matter what, though, don't drink coffee on an empty stomach. The caffeine in coffee triggers cortisol levels to rise. Coffee is also an appetite suppressant, which can work against regular meals and blood sugar balance.

Also note that a medication can be toxic if it is not the right one for you or the dose is too high and your body cannot clear it easily, causing it to build up in your system.

9. **For weight loss, aim to match the amount you eat (your "fuel") to your activity level—before you expend energy.** If your activity is higher in the morning, make sure your breakfast supplies the fuel for that. If most of your activity is in the afternoon or both morning and afternoon, then lunch should provide enough fuel for your upcoming energy expenditure. Dinner isn't typically as important for building up your energy—unless you go night skiing! At dinnertime, you'll still want protein and vegetables, because vegetables provide important nutrients, but you don't necessarily need anything starchy at the end of the day.

10. **Take a few basic vitamins and supplements for a healthy foundation, and develop a longer-term, personalized plan.** I know from experience that taking a bunch of supplements willy-nilly will not improve your health. It's all too easy to get seduced by magazine ads, store displays, and the latest thing your friend is trying. Most "experts" and websites are trying to sell you something, no matter how well intentioned. The FDA does not regulate supplements, unlike medications, and their quality varies, so do your research and make sure the supplements you take are really what you need (ideally in consultation with a knowledgeable nutritionist).

Personalized vitamins are something I've tried and like because the vitamins are built to supplement the deficiencies my blood tests reveal. My nutritionist helps me do this and it costs about $300 for a four-month supply, which is not much more than regular vitamins. My blood is tested every three months and the vitamins are reconfigured after each test to meet my body's changing needs. If you'd like to try this, work with a nutritionist who uses personalized vitamins to help his or her patients.

When you take this approach, it likely will change your life, as it has mine and so many others. A friend of mine is a perfect example. She hadn't been feeling well for most of a year. She had never been a complainer, but when I'd see her she'd mention she was having bouts of nausea or upsetting blurry vision and mental fogginess, and she was tired constantly. She had the scare of her life when she thought she passed out briefly while driving. Her doctor ordered tons of tests and blood work, looking for hepatitis, abdominal cancers, and lots more she didn't want to think about. Everything came back negative, except she was low in iron. My friend began iron shots and felt a little better but was still not feeling well.

I finally convinced her to see a nutritionist with an integrative approach, who ran a complete nutritional panel on her. It came back with indications that she was deficient in more than two dozen vitamins and minerals. Working with the nutritionist, she started changing her diet and taking targeted supplements in addition to multivitamins, which she never thought she needed. The biggest sign of her recovery is that she's not thinking about how bad she feels every day. It's more occasional and her energy and comfort is increasing week by week.

The key to reaping the benefits of this personalized approach to supplements is getting blood tests every quarter in an effort to see how your nutrient balance is affected by such things as seasonal changes, stress, and diet. Each vitamin and mineral is like an instrument in an orchestra that works in harmony with the others, constantly changing to blend with the whole. The lab then creates the vitamin and mineral compounds specific to your needs and calculates how the supplements interact to get just the right balance.

11. **In the same week, get your blood tested by your general practitioner and a nutritionist.** I do this three to four times a year. The reason? Conventional labs run high-level tests that insurance covers and, in some cases, only begins indicating abnormal results when a disease has already taken hold. Results from the tests my nutritionist runs act as a check and balance to the traditional system. By analyzing my micronutrient levels, I can take specific actions to treat deficiencies and ward off disease before it sets in. Testing by both practitioners in the same week means I get to review results influenced by similar foods and similar amounts of stress and activity.

A QUICK INTRODUCTION
TO A BASELINE OF VITAMINS

As a starting point, whether you're dealing with specific health issues or are focused on maximizing your healthy edge, there is a baseline of vitamins and supplements that *do* matter to all of us at midlife. They support the foundation of a strong immune system, gut health, and the management of inflammation.

B12. A deficiency of vitamin B12 can develop, especially in people over age 50 and in vegans. Levels can be easily checked with a blood test. It's important for brain and muscle function and mostly comes from animal protein foods, but is not always well absorbed by the body.

Fish oil (Omega–3 fatty acids). Unless you eat fish three or more times a week, you should consider taking a fish oil supplement. Fish oil is anti-inflammatory and helps with many other functions of the body.

If you do eat fish regularly, concerns about mercury mean you need to be very picky about the types and amounts of fish you consume. The recommendation is to "think small" in terms of fish size, and look at the information labels in the fish department of your market. Try sardines, flounder, haddock, salmon, and trout. Either avoid swordfish, tuna, and halibut or eat them less than three times a month. The NRDC (National Resource Defense Council) has an excellent guide. There is also a phone app called Seafood Watch by the Monterey Bay Aquarium that rates fish based both on overfishing and toxicity.

A daily probiotic. A good probiotic helps maintain a healthy environment for your gut. Oral probiotics are beneficial bacteria that supplement the microbes already in your digestive system. Choose one with multiple strains.

Curcumin. Curcumin is a constituent of the spice turmeric, which is known to reduce inflammation. Turmeric is found in curry and other Indian foods, and you can take turmeric supplements to get your curcumin. Curcumin has been studied in hundreds of published articles and is something that can be taken safely daily.

Green tea. A potent antioxidant, a good-quality organic green tea can really enhance your well-being.

A caution about vitamin C. Vitamin C has ascorbic acid in it, which is very tough on your stomach lining. If you have Chron's disease, diverticulitis, or any kind of intestinal problems and you take those large chewable vitamin Cs, especially in megadoses, it can actually tear your stomach lining up. Be cautious and discuss with your doctor.

A Caution about calcium. Make sure you are tested for your calcium level before taking supplements. Studies are showing that getting calcium from calcium-rich foods is preferable to getting calcium from supplements. Foods rich in calcium include fat-free milk (available lactose-free) and other dairy products—which are all options if you eat dairy—and foods like broccoli, sardines, salmon, and dark green leafy vegetables. Talk to your doctor about how much calcium you are typically eating in a day and whether that is enough for you, taking into account whether you are at risk for fractures.

Vitamin vacations. I've been advised to take vitamin vacations so my body does not become too dependent on supplementation.

In the past, I would eat something like 3,500 calories a day. Today, it's more like 1,900 and less than 400 at dinner—though I don't count calories.

I cut out almost all foods with added sugars. I cut down my protein to four- or five-ounce (palm-sized) portions. (Many of you may need to increase your protein if you've been avoiding it.) I doubled or tripled the amounts of fresh, raw, or lightly cooked vegetables I eat. To encourage cell replenishment, I make super foods part of my daily diet. This includes foods like eggs, spinach, broccoli, avocados, and green tea. I don't feel hungry and I'm not thinking about food all the time. More healthful foods have taken away all that urgency—physical and mental—that I used to feel about food.

I still have treats, but they're real treats—small amounts I eat on occasion, not regularly, and most often in the company of friends and family. I have a growing appreciation for food as a social experience that feeds our need for connection, relaxation, and slowing down.

Most of all, I've come to understand that what and how we eat is a lifestyle choice: we can eat "killing foods" or we can consume nourishing, life- and cell-enhancing foods. From that vantage point, healthy eating becomes, literally, a self-fulfilling way of being. Your body also becomes more pure and will let you know it's unhappy when you eat unhealthy foods. Check in with your body after you eat your favorite bad food and see if you have a headache, stomachache, gas, or tiredness. Once you make this connection, you won't want that food much anymore.

Your Healthy Edge

DEVELOPING YOUR CURIOSITY AND HEALTH KNOWLEDGE

DEVELOPING YOUR EATING HABITS

Food has a massive impact on your health, especially as you age. Below are some ideas you can put into practice to help give your body a chance to detoxify, heal, and feel wonderful!

- ☐ Take one full hour to eat dinner once each week.

- ☐ Remove all added sugar from your diet for 30 days. Note your weight, blood sugar, and blood pressure at the beginning of this experiment and at the end. Journal each day, describing how you feel and any changes you notice in your mood, gut health, energy levels, and cravings.

- ☐ Remove all dairy from your diet for 30 days. Note your weight and blood pressure at the beginning of this experiment and at the end. Journal each day, describing how you feel and any changes you notice in your mood, gut health, energy levels, and cravings.

- ☐ Follow the eating guidelines in this book for 30 days. Note your weight and blood pressure at the beginning of this experiment and at the end. Journal each day, describing how you feel and any changes you notice in your mood, energy levels, and cravings.

- ☐ Fast for 12 hours each day between dinner and breakfast to give your body a chance to repair and detoxify.

■ Drink water. Multiply your weight by two-thirds. That number is the total number of ounces you should drink each day. Note: If you weigh more than 200 pounds, check with your doctor about the amount of water you should drink each day.

■ Make an appointment with a nutritionist who can customize a food and supplement plan to meet your body's specific needs.

Don't Stop the Music

CONTINUOUS MOVEMENT STRENGTHENS YOUR INNER TREE OF LIFE

"Exercise should be regarded
as a tribute to the heart."

—GENE TUNNEY, BOXER

Over the last several decades natural movement in our everyday lives has dwindled significantly. I believe that this decrease in movement is a root cause of many of the health problems we face today. I also know there is a lot we can do about it, and the effort doesn't have to be hard. Inside this chapter I ask you to:

- Think about moving your body rather than exercising. Find ways to incorporate more natural movement into your day, rather than thinking you need to do aggressive exercise to be healthy.

- Understand the impacts the abundance of sitting and technology has on your health and how you can counteract it.

- Consider the benefits your limbs, organs, brain, and capillaries reap by providing them with fresh blood supply through movement.

- Learn how movement improves your mood and relieves depression and anxiety.

I didn't put the word *exercise* in this chapter title because I'm biased against it. Exercise connotes something many people don't want to do. It's something unnatural and it sounds a bit like medicine. I want to promote the idea of *movement.* It's what our bodies naturally do.

In my parents' generation people moved their bodies as a normal part of their everyday routines, without thinking about it as "exercise." They walked to the bank or the post office, where they often had to stand in line for a while. If they wanted to learn something, they walked over to the encyclopedia on the bookshelf or went to the library, where they browsed the aisles, sat down at a table, and got up to browse some more. For fun, they often went dancing. I remember my mother going dancing well into her 80s.

We don't do most of those things anymore. We think, "I'm much more active than my dad, because I go to the gym five days a week. My dad never went to the gym."

My so-called "girlfriend" Dolly (yes, my wife approves) lives in Napa at one of our Aegis communities. She's 104. I adore her because she is so humorous and optimistic. I call her and send her flowers on her birthday. On her recent birthday I said, "Dolly, you have to tell me your secret." With her earnest and commanding voice, she said, "I never sit down and I always have a project!"

A rapper friend of mine wrote lyrics that speak to what Dolly's generation has that we need to regain. It's that sense of determination to do what's good for us. The lyrics say:

> I wanna get exercise, but I'm too lazy to work out
> I want all the finer things, but don't wanna go to work now
> I wanna go outside, take my family to the beach
> I wake up in the morning, first thing I do is look at a screen, at a screen

My friend is right, and I laugh when I hear people my age or younger say that they will live much longer than their parents because they are in the gym all the time and their dad never worked out. I say, "Really? Do you handwash your car? Do your own laundry? Mow your own lawn? Walk your dog?" The point is that the generation that came before mine got much more natural movement every day. The dad I'm talking about got about 12,000 to 14,000 steps a day just by living his life. We can do the same.

Epidemiologist Alpa Patel, PhD, at the American Cancer Society, describes a type of person that is common in lots of circles—the "active couch potato." As she explains, "This person goes to the gym and maintains a healthy weight, but spends the majority of the rest of their time in sedentary activities—sitting at work, in the car, and at home."

You really have to think beyond the 30 minutes a day in which you're intentionally engaging in physical activity. What does the rest of your day look like? Do you mow your lawn? When was the last time you got up to use a phone book? When I was a kid, we probably went to the phone book three times a day to look up a number, and we raced to the phone to answer it.

At Aegis, most of our residents have never been to a gym, which only came into vogue in the 1960s with Gold's Gym and the fame of Jack LaLanne (who at one time was a spokesperson for Aegis) and later in 1982 with Jane Fonda's "feel the burn" workout videos. If you ask our residents about their exercise habits, they think about pastimes and sports like skiing, baseball, or dancing. In Europe it can still be hard to find a gym. People bike and walk—to the store, to town, to take a stroll with friends and family. They play soccer and boccie everywhere there.

In our *"age of the device"*—my term—moving our bodies isn't required anymore because everything we need is right at our smartphone fingertips. We have remotes for every device and we even text each other when we're in different rooms. There are even people who are replacing their lawns with pretty gravel, not so much to save water and help the environment but to avoid the physical work and upkeep of a yard.

All that sitting shows up in our cells, our cell longevity, and our total wellness. It's another example of the sandpile effect: we're either adding to the pile of sand that is holding up the stick (our bodies), or we're eroding the sand and making the stick (ourselves) vulnerable to falling over. We're either weakening or strengthening our healthy edge.

We need to get moving.

Sitting Is the New Smoking: The Medical Consequences of Inactivity

The first time I heard the phrase "sitting is the new smoking," a light bulb went off. "That's it!" I said to myself.

After years of studying our increasingly sedentary lifestyles, James Levine, MD, PhD, director of the Mayo Clinic/Arizona State University Obesity Solutions Initiative, put it this way in his book *Get Up!*: "Sitting is more dangerous than smoking …. It kills more people than HIV and is more treacherous than parachuting. We are sitting ourselves to death."

That is not a metaphor. While smoking rates have decreased, sitting rates are rising. According to current estimates, 5.3 million people die due to causes related to inactivity and a sedentary lifestyle compared with about 5 million who die from smoking. Studies repeatedly show that the effects of long-term sitting include health risks like weight gain, cholesterol problems, heart disease, type 2 diabetes, and greater susceptibility to falls and broken bones.

I was shocked to discover that even parenting and grandparenting, which once involved large expenditures of energetic activity, no longer do. When the Mayo Clinic studied the activity levels of mothers of school-age kids, they tracked both physical activity (cooking, cleaning, playing with children, and exercising) and sedentary time (in front of televisions, tablets, computers, and driving). They found that over the past 50 years, sedentary time has increased by seven hours a week, and physical activity has decreased by 11 hours a week. I would go so far as to say that "technology is the new cancer"—the impact is silent and epidemic. It's changing our lifestyle habits in ways that are pervasive and detrimental.

> "SITTING IS MORE DANGEROUS THAN SMOKING …. IT KILLS MORE PEOPLE THAN HIV AND IS MORE TREACHEROUS THAN PARACHUTING. WE ARE SITTING OURSELVES TO DEATH."
>
> — James Levine, MD, PhD, director of the Mayo Clinic/Arizona State University Obesity Solutions Initiative

The difference between sitting—that is, being sedentary—and movement is critical. We know from many studies of the past decade that bursts of exercise several times a week is not counterweight to the risks of not moving.

When I was a young administrator at an assisted living residence in Montana, there was a resident I really enjoyed who was confined to a wheelchair. One day she came into my office and said:

> When I was 6 years old, all I wanted to do was to ride on my grandpa's horse. My dad would say, "You should walk, you'll always need those legs." When I was 19, all I wanted to do was to ride in my boyfriend's Ford coupe and my dad would say, "You should walk, you'll always need those legs." When I married and had kids, my dream was to ride on an airplane and although my father had passed away by the time I took my first plane ride, I could hear his voice say, "You should walk, you'll always need those legs." Now I'm 83 and confined to a wheelchair and all I dream of is walking. I guess I needed those legs.

When we don't move continuously throughout the day, we're jeopardizing our health—we're literally cutting short the lives of our cells. It's time we started thinking about movement, not exercise, and develop our habits of health to include things as simple as walking, standing, and not sitting.

The London Bus Conductor Effect

A 1953 study showed that bus conductors in London, who walked up and down the length and up and down the stairs of their double-decker buses, had half the number of deaths from coronary heart disease than did the bus drivers who spent their day sitting at the wheel. This was the first study to recognize a link between physical activity and health outcomes.

The Midlife Turning Point

The sitting effect is exacerbated with age. For example, our skeletal muscle mass—those muscles that attach to your bones—start to deteriorate. That's why we begin to look flabby and gravity takes its toll on every part of our bodies. It also explains all the jokes about gravity, like "everything seems to go down."

That aging cliff we talked about earlier really hits us physically between the ages of 50 and 70, when we lose about 30% of our strength. We lose another 30% each decade that follows. Muscle mass also declines with age. Sedentary habits can be compared to the extreme version of inactivity. For example, for every day spent in bed, studies show you can lose 1% of muscle strength. At the same time, we're losing muscle mass in midlife—meaning our muscles don't repair themselves as quickly as they used to—and we're getting stiffer and our tissues are less able to tolerate stress.

These declines happen much more quickly and severely if we're more sedentary than if we're active. As soon as we become less sedentary, the aging process can be slowed and even reversed. There's a simple prescription: *move*.

Here's a great example. My wife, T, and I took the grandkids school shopping and after four hours we came home. I looked at my Fitbit at 7 pm and said, "We need to go for a walk." It looked like we hadn't had any exercise all day. I had only 4,687 steps on my Fitbit, but when T checked hers, it had 11,678 steps! How could this be? We were glued at the hip all day, never more than a few feet apart.

Or so I thought.

So we retraced the day's events. When we went to the store, I sat in the comfy couch of the shoe department. Meanwhile, T told me that she'd paced back and forth, helping the grandkids shop. She turned over nearly every shoe in that store for an hour. When we went to look at kids clothes, I leaned against a rack and checked e-mails while she checked out every item on every rack for 90 minutes. While our grandson went to try stuff on in the dressing room for 30 minutes, I went in with him while T went around the store and brought items to us. These little habits add up—she more than doubled my Fitbit output while still being within shouting distance, just a few feet away.

Another example is cooking. I love cooking dinner and can easily add 3,000 steps to my daily total just by doing something I love to do. My belief about step counting and what's the right amount is that the more steps you can do each day the better. The trick is to not make the steps seem like steps. For me, it's taking a walk in the morning and one in the evening after dinner. The rest of my steps I get from living life. This way, getting steps is just part of my day and you can make it part of yours too without it being daunting. Remember to track it. Write it down. The more you see what you did, the more likely you are to improve your number.

Bottom line: You don't have to run five miles away from home to get exercise; just go school shopping with my wife. Though I didn't know it at the time, I made taking steps a spectator sport. So while I am not saying you need to run to be healthy, I do believe interval training is important for heart health. While you are walking, make sure to add in climbing stairs and hills or moving the treadmill to an incline to get your heart rate up for a few minutes. Do this off and on while you are getting your steps in.

Dr. Mimi Guarneri, the world-leading expert on heart health and president of the Academy of Integrative Health and Medicine, explains: "We are more than our genes. Even genetic predispositions can be altered by something as simple as walking. Research shows that your genes are not your destiny. Your genes require an environment in which to interact."

Thus, while you may have the genes for obesity, for example, you may never develop obesity if you are like the Amish community that was studied by the University of Maryland. The Amish carry the obesity gene (a mutation called the FTO gene), but because they walk 18,000 steps a day, they aren't obese, as was reported in the *Archives of Internal Medicine*. In the study, physical activity was even more significant than diet in maintaining their health. They've protected their people from type 2 diabetes through their work habits and lifestyle, which are all based on movement—walking and manual labor rather than driving and technology.

> FOR THE AMISH, PHYSICAL ACTIVITY WAS EVEN MORE SIGNIFICANT THAN DIET IN MAINTAINING THEIR HEALTH. THEY'VE PROTECTED THEIR PEOPLE FROM TYPE 2 DIABETES THROUGH THEIR WORK HABITS AND LIFESTYLE, WHICH ARE ALL BASED ON MOVEMENT—WALKING AND MANUAL LABOR RATHER THAN DRIVING AND TECHNOLOGY.

The study revealed something else: population-wide obesity is a modern phenomenon. Like the Amish, we carry the same genes our ancestors did. What this means is that our lifestyle changes—such as sitting too much and poor diets—have brought on the obesity and diabetes epidemics.

How we live our lives and the environment we live it in are the determinants of our health and longevity, with genes being just one important factor. If the environment encourages us to remain seated while a device does the work, we need to think about changing our environment to move more and sit less.

Movement Versus Exercise

Without exercise, muscles will atrophy—or at least that is what people have been taught. There's a problem with that bit of wisdom. It is not exercise per se that prevents atrophy and lifestyle-based aging. It's *movement*.

Back to my car analogies: You buy a car and say, "This is a great vehicle. I'm going to keep it in the garage for three years and never start it or move it." What's going to happen? The battery is going to die right away. The tires are going to disintegrate. The seals will rot. The metal will rust. The same thing happens to us. If we don't move, we rust. We start to corrode from inside.

> "FIND A PLACE OF HAPPY ENERGY, OR HAPPY EXERTION."
>
> — Dr. Becky Su

So what kind of movement do we need? Many of us think we need to work all the machines in the gym or play fast pickup basketball on Fridays or do step aerobics class a few times a week. Those might meet current guidelines for aerobic activities, but that doesn't address our need to stop our sedentary patterns.

I especially believe we have to stop seeing exercise as synonymous with running—lots of running, whether it's the treadmill or training and running a half or full marathon. Based on data from 3,800 men and women over the age of 35, The American College of Cardiology recently found that runners who average more than 20 miles a week don't live as long as those who run less than 20 miles a week. On average, the long-distance runners lived about as long as people who didn't run much at all.

The conclusion I draw is that our bodies are designed to be moved in a continuous way, but not overworked and overstressed. You can't take a Ferrari on a 150-mile-an-hour thrill ride on an old country road every day.

I've had too many friends keel over and wind up in the hospital because they pushed themselves with their running, biking, or workouts but weren't taking care of everything else. You can be healthy—even healthier—if you don't push your heart rate to 150 or 160 beats per minute every time you work out. Just do some interval training to get your heart rate up and back down several times while getting your steps in.

Dr. Becky Su, the master of both Western and Chinese medicine and acupuncture whom you met earlier in the book, thinks we need to get much more assertive about the harm of "aggressive exercise." She wants people to find a place of "happy energy, or happy exertion." For most of us, pushing ourselves too hard can push our bodies beyond their normal ability to repair.

Dr. Su explains, "People who say they feel sick if they can't run and are used to their 'runner's high' are actually describing the effect of withdrawal from their own hormones. It's like taking a drug."

Researchers who study centenarians (people who live more than 100 years) pretty much discover that none of them "work out." Most of these elders have never seen a gym. They don't know what a trainer is. They don't lift weights or run marathons. Journalist Dan Buettner spent five years in partnership with the National Geographic Society studying individuals who are 90 or even 100 years old and are living active, relatively healthy lives without medication all the way to the very end. He identified their communities as Blue Zones and his books, including *The Blue Zones Solution,* are inspiring.

The "exercise" habits he identified are simple: walking, gardening and farming, climbing stairs and hillsides, and household chores, all of which they routinely do for more than five hours a day every day. What these centenarians share is a lifestyle that includes frequent and gentle exercise as part of their daily lives. Their movements are natural—the things the body does without contorting itself or putting excessive pressure on any single part.

These are not just special cases but examples of cultures in which people are, as Buettner puts it, "exercising mindlessly." Or as Dr. Su would say, "They don't run themselves ragged," putting the emphasis on the word "run."

Circulation: Our Inner Tree of Life

Shirley Newell, MD, chief medical officer at Aegis Living, explains why your body always needs to move, especially as it ages. It comes down to good circulation. "If your hands and feet are cold, the solution is to get out and exercise, not to put on gloves or stand in front of the heater. When you stand up suddenly on a hot day and you pass out, it's because the blood is pooled to your extremities."

A young body has a heart that is pumping at full velocity.

When you get older, it takes more effort to circulate your blood through your vascular tree, which runs throughout every part of your body to the tips of your fingers and toes. Your vascular system just isn't as smooth, efficient, and powerful as it once was.

You can think of the body as being like a tree with an image of a sturdy trunk, larger branches, smaller and smaller branches, and a spray of leaves. In the body, oxygen flows from the lungs to the heart (trunk), to the great arterial vessels (large branches), into the smaller vessels, arteries, and arterioles (smaller branches), and into the capillaries (leaves). The oxygen is extracted from the capillaries where it feeds the tissues, and then the deoxygenated blood is exchanged at the capillary level. All the deoxygenated blood, with its carbon dioxide and waste, is carried away through the venous tree back to the lungs, where it is reoxygenated and recirculated through the heart. Keeping the circulatory system functioning well and having good flow and exchange down to the microvascular level is essential.

Microcirculation allows blood flow in the smaller arteries, arterioles, and capillaries that supply individual cells. This is where real health happens. This is not just for your lungs and extremities. Likewise, the microvasculature of your brain is critical to preserving brain function and cognition. Many believe that poor circulation and damage to the microcirculation are a central issue in dementia.

Good joint and spinal health relies on movement that provides a fresh blood supply and the removal of toxins. As we age, the cells that make up this system actually begin to break down, but exercise helps to maintain and restore the microvascular circulation.

From an Eastern perspective, this circulation system and tree of life is part of the chi—or life force. It's the movement of energy that flows through us, and all things.

It is essential to get blood to flow into your capularies–your fingertips and toes for example. You can do this through basic movement, yoga, stretching, and massage. I tell my friends there is a functional reason for massage. It isn't just to feel good. It's so capillaries don't die. It gets blood into them so all parts of your body benefit, even your brain.

Movement and exercise aren't about bigger muscles. It's not about being more beautiful. It's not so you can run an eight-minute mile. It's to enhance the flow through your circulatory tree, your strength and flexibility, and maintain your brain, bones, and moods.

Basically I'm talking about the typical tortoise-and-the-hare scenario. We want to be there at the end. That's the point. As Americans we have it wrong. We say we want to do the big, hard things. But that's not really what we want.

We want to be healthy for a long time, to walk a mile in our 80s, and be able to toss our grandkids in the air. We want endurance.

Forest Bathing: Take an Easy Walk Under the Trees

I knew being in nature was good for me, but recently I learned the science behind why. I recently watched a video on the World Economic Forum's website about Japanese forest bathing, or Shinrin-yoku. Shinrin-yoku means "spending more time around trees," and it was launched as a national Japanese health program in 1982. There are no heavy-duty workouts required, just quiet contemplation around trees. Japan has been studying the physical and psychological effects of forest bathing and learned that along with the health benefits of fresh air, the trees emit oils as protection from germs and insects. These oils are called phytoncides and they help our immune systems. Studies found that forests lower blood pressure and reduce stress hormones and depression, all while boosting energy. Forests are turning out to be a healing balm for urban children and for those wanting to escape technology. It's like our grandparents used to say: "Get outside and get some fresh air!" They were right. Regular contact with nature really does improve well-being.

The Brain: Work the Body, Work the Mind

As we age, our synapses—the connections between nerve cells (neurons)—break down or are destroyed. The hippocampus, that area of the brain that controls learning and memory formation, also begins to shrink. Chemicals called neurotransmitters, which relay signals between neurons, diminish. Beyond any doubt, physical exercise, no matter when it is begun, can slow down these changes.

There's actually a protein called BDNF—brain-derived neurotrophic factor—that supports the growth of existing brain cells and the development of new ones. At least in the lab, exercise produces higher levels of BDNF in mice, with exciting implications for humans. Movement increases the number of synapses, stimulates the brain to develop more neurons in the hippocampus, and may also help integrate new neurons into the brain's wiring.

Since the fear of Alzheimer's disease weighs on all our minds, there is good news on the relationship of exercise to memory and many studies are underway. In fact, many experts are coming to believe that vascular impairment may be more of a factor than Alzheimer's disease in the surge of dementia related to aging. Though it was once thought that brain damage due to strokes was permanent, greater understanding of brain plasticity is disproving that belief.

One researcher, Teresa Liu-Ambrose, PhD, PT, of the University of British Columbia, looked at people with vascular-related cognitive impairment—that's the common form of memory loss caused by problems with blood flow to the brain usually due to stroke or small vessel disease. These processes are known as ministrokes, or TIAs (transient ischemic attacks), which become more common over the age of 55 but can occur at any age. In her small study, participants who walked outdoors for 40 minutes three times a week over six months showed noticeable improvements on memory tests, compared with a control group that was sedentary.

Walk Your Heart: Pump Your Vital Muscle

Our minds might worry us the most, but our hearts can take our lives away without warning. For a long time research on heart health and the role of exercise focused on intense cardio workouts. In the 1990s researchers began looking at the benefits of smaller amounts of activity.

According to I-Min Lee, MD, MPH, ScD, of Harvard Medical School, "The research backs up what we all know intuitively: Almost any amount of regular exercise promotes longevity. Even small amounts of exercise can make a big difference."

One study of 55,000 adults showed that running just five to 10 minutes a day reduced mortality from all causes by 30% and from cardiovascular disease by 45%—adding up to three years to a person's life span. A Harvard study analyzing more than 33 studies (what's known as a *meta-analysis*) specifically evaluated the role of exercise and the risk for coronary heart disease. It found that people who exercised moderately 150 minutes a week (or 20-30 minutes per day) had a 14% lower risk compared with those who were totally inactive. If you double that number of minutes, it found, the risk is 20% lower.

While on our most recent vacation to Italy we spent several glorious days on the island of Capri. It's our sixth visit here, so clearly we love it. Our favorite hotel sits partway up the massive hill that overlooks the harbor and is adjacent to the steep stairs that lead to the center of the village at the top of the hill. The first morning, I looked out the window and happened to notice a woman walking up the stairs who was wrapped in wintery garb that made her stand out in such a hot, sunny place.

The stairs are maybe a 30% grade going up. I lost track of her and turned my attention to the boats below. But then, on our second day, I noticed her again as I looked out the window. I was intrigued. On the third day, I kept my eyes peeled, and sure enough, I saw the same woman all wrapped up in the 85-degree heat.

On an impulse I laced up my sneakers and sprinted to catch up with her. I saw her come out of a little store holding a small container of milk. As I gasped to catch my breath, I went into the store to ask the proprietor if she knew the lady I saw every day. "Yes," she said, and continued in broken English, "She come every day. Don't like milk. Just like the walking." It turned out the woman would give the milk away to someone she passed along the way. Every day she made the 30- or 40-minute walk to the top of Capri and back. She was over 90 years old and had that purpose to move every day, climbing like she was half her age.

> "ALMOST ANY AMOUNT OF REGULAR EXERCISE PROMOTES LONGEVITY. EVEN SMALL AMOUNTS OF EXERCISE CAN MAKE A BIG DIFFERENCE."
>
> — I-Min Lee, Harvard Medical School

If you are out of shape and thinking 150 to 300 minutes a week is too much, here's some news that will help you at least start to move more and get your heart pumping. A Taiwanese study looked at people who smoked, drank heavily, or had diabetes, all of which put them at risk for heart disease, and found they had a 14% lower risk for dying if they averaged just 15 minutes of low activity a day.

I always tell people that while most types of exercise are beneficial, the type that works best is the one that you will actually do.

Bone Health: Stay Standing

You can have a healthy heart and no memory problems, but if you're going to fall and break your hip, it may well be curtains. Why?

Bones are what hold us up. Good balance is what keeps us from falling and, in many cases, keeps us from dying.

Let's reverse-engineer what happens. If we work backward from old age, many people ultimately die of immune deficiencies and associated diseases like pneumonia. How do they get pneumonia? I have seen this over and over. They fall and they don't get out of bed because they are incapacitated. Then they may get a respiratory infection that evolves into pneumonia. Even if you are healthy, after age 65 a hip fracture increases your chance of death over the next year threefold (you'll learn more on how to prevent that later).

Many people don't know that they have bad bones until they actually injure themselves. If they fall and experience a hip fracture or some other structural injury, their health becomes tenuous. There are lots of risk factors, but one of the best ways to improve or stabilize bone density is by doing weight-bearing exercise or yoga, which has the added benefits of reducing stress and inflammation and improving immune function. These activities also increase muscle strength, which improves stability and protects the bones.

Emotions: A Life in Balance

You might not realize it, but the movement habit has an extra benefit: it supports healthy mood. How we feel emotionally is as important to our health and longevity as how we feel physically. Experts have long confirmed that physical activity helps relieve depression, anxiety, and stress at every stage of life, but it is especially important as we get older. This is a case of good habits supporting good habits: movement supports good mood and good mood gets you off the couch and moving around.

In a culture where 11% of people use antidepressants and where the risk of becoming dependent on these medications is high among people in their older years, we have to acknowledge—and act on the fact—that exercise can be as effective a treatment for those with mild to major depression and can have longer-lasting results. Even better, moderate exercise may also help prevent depression.

Recently Duke University ran a trial with people over 50 who felt depressed. One group took an aerobic exercise class for 16 weeks. The comparison group just took an antidepressant medication. The result: the exercise class, according to participants, was as effective as the medication in improving mood.

Much of this relief comes because when your body is moving, your brain is increasing its production of neurotransmitters such as serotonin, dopamine, and norepinephrine—the very neurotransmitters targeted by drug treatments. One specific neurotransmitter, called GABA, that when activated, helps calm brain activity and minimizes anxiety.

Aerobic exercise in particular seems to substantially increase the production of new brain cells in the brain's hippocampus, which is involved in controlling emotions and processing memories, along with other functions. Aerobic exercise may lessen the rumination, or obsessive negative thinking, that is one of the hallmarks of depression and anxiety.

Last, but surely not least, regular exercise improves body image and self-esteem. It is depressing to think we have to accept our "midlife muffin tops," the struggle to climb several flights of stairs without running out of breath, or our lack of strength when we want to carry and lift things—like overhead luggage. A healthy approach to movement changes us from the inside out, like all the habits of health. It can also protect mood and help us reinforce our sense of connection to others, which is important for health and happiness.

GirlTrek: Women Who Walk, Talk, and Empower Themselves

One of the best examples of the power of movement to generate positive emotions is what happened with a group called GirlTrek. It started when two women who wanted to get healthier by walking together teamed up to meet their goal. Their first steps led to the founding of the organization called GirlTrek. Its mission is to inspire black women to change their lives and communities by walking. The cornerstone activities of GirlTrek are 10-week group walking challenges that emphasize the rewards of taking time for yourself, getting outside, and connecting with others in a nonjudgmental and noncompetitive way.

As David Bornstein wrote in a *New York Times* article called "Walking Together for Health and Spirit":

"They don't talk about looking good, but about looking alive: having the 'GirlTrek glow.' They inspire women with images of courage and dignity …. They encourage women to think of their health as a community service; they celebrate trekkers when they reach goals and milestones. They encourage new traditions — a family walk after the Thanksgiving dinner, a ritual of walking the kids to school."

The founders of GirlTrek are aware of a rich cultural history of walking in their communities—from traveling on foot to freedom during the days of slavery to marching for civil rights. As they walk, they remember this history and their brave ancestors.

The thousands of women who participate in the GirlTrek movement are reaping lasting rewards from their walking: deep conversation and friendship along with physical health benefits including weight loss, reduced risk factors for disease, better emotional health, and healthier children, who often join their moms and aunts on the walks.

The Ancient Practice of Qigong for Modern Times

No matter how much movement we add into our daily lives, we can enhance our natural movements with the ancient approach of mindful exercise—the inner art of movement. The Chinese practices of qigong and tai chi focus on "the mind leading the body," Dr. Su teaches. With these practices, you don't look in the mirror to do it the "right" way. There's no way to do the movements and sequences "perfectly." Everyone is different and the movement comes from the inside, where each of us is unique.

Qigong and other movement practices are believed to stimulate the liver, pancreas, and lungs with subtle, gentle movement and simultaneously connect the body and the brain, improve our balance, and enhance flexibility. These flowing movement practices even build strength because you hold positions and work with the natural weight of the body. But there's no gasping for air or pushing yourself to reach a target goal. Qigong is not a struggle, a fight, or a contest. There are no titans of war here. Qigong is not a weekend warrior activity; it's a part of life.

We have a fascinating natural research experiment within our own Aegis Living communities. Our first culturally specific assisted living community, Aegis Gardens, founded in 2001, was designed for the large number of Chinese families in Fremont, California, who were asking for ways to provide a greater sense of home—from food to decor to activities—for their older relatives, something we know is a leading factor in extending the everyday engagement and functioning of our residents.

In our Chinese community, we began to notice something: the residents in this community seemed to be living longer than non-Chinese residents. We wondered if it was their primarily vegetarian diet or maybe the fact that they meditated. We looked at our data on falls, but they weren't definitive either. When we discussed the phenomenon with our Aegis Gardens staff, we realized that while our Chinese residents had falls, they were experiencing far fewer falls requiring hospitalization. It's well known that a lengthy hospitalization for a broken hip (or anything else) can lead to rapid decline and even death. What was responsible for the reduced number of falls—particularly serious ones?

One thing we know is that most of our Chinese residents take classes in qigong or do some form healing movement every day. Qigong means "life energy cultivation". It's a holistic system of postures, movement, breathing, and meditation. The largest benefit of qigong is that it helps with circulation, which we've seen is the best weapon against atrophy—that means better balance and greater strength.

The classes at Aegis Garden also teach something called a "soft drop": when you feel yourself falling, you roll with it. Athletes know this, and it seems to be instinctual when people have been practicing the flowing movements of qigong or tai chi. The slow drop's rolling movement prevents one part of the body from taking all the pressure of the body's weight when we fall. The number one way people die in the hospital is due to the aftermath of a fall. Death from a fall is typically a result of pneumonia that fall victims contract. They get pneumonia because they are on their backs recovering and aren't using their lungs properly. It's true most people will recover from a fall, but it can be very hard to get back to the previous state of health.

What is the root cause of falls? It gets back to balance and other factors, which are exacerbated by dehydration.

My Practices for Balance and Flow

In addition to my habit of constant hydration, I like to stand on one leg while brushing my teeth or watching TV. I'm also a huge proponent of both qigong and tai chi because both involve constant gentle flowing motions, like a wave or a bird in flight. The movements imitate nature in many ways: the ebb and flow of waves in a lake or ocean and the movements of animals, birds, snakes, or butterflies. One of the best qigong exercises is called "Big Bird," where you put your arms all the way out and slowly move them up and down, almost like you have wings. You can actually feel the blood moving through your body and feeding into the tips of your fingers, promoting microcirculation.

"Steps" and Tips for
More Movement and Less Sitting

1. **Set goals and track your daily steps.**

   Many studies of the benefits of movement are limited because they rely on self-reporting—"I walked for two miles, and I only watched TV for one hour" —which is notoriously unreliable. One of the most important things you can do right now is begin to measure your actual activity, starting with tracking how many steps you take from the moment you wake up in the morning.

If you do nothing during the day but sit on the couch or at a computer and you only get up to go to the bathroom, you may take about 2,500 to 3,000 steps a day. At less than 5,000 steps daily, your body will atrophy. It takes very roughly that many steps a day to maintain weight, health, and fitness.

The American Heart Association recommends 10,000 steps a day. The more the better—just remember the Amish. I try to trick myself into getting the steps I need. I try to get about 5,000 steps before 9 am by taking a long walk with my dog, doing an exercise routine, or doing some other combination of activity. Then my daily routines will get me to 10,000 steps without much conscious effort. If I don't get that number due to a packed meeting schedule or something else, then I make sure I'm the one cooking. I can get 3,000 steps moving around the kitchen and cleaning up and then a few more steps with an after-dinner walk. A CEO friend of mine does it another way. He gets exercise into his busy day by scheduling all his staff calls during the first two hours of the morning, while he's on his walk.

The main message is to set goals and measure, and always remember that some is good and more (within your own limits) is better.

2. Minimize—and track—sitting time.

While an antisitting movement isn't yet in place, it's time to start your own. In addition to tracking your daily steps, spend several days tracking the amount of time you spend sitting—or lounging. Use a timer and record all your inactivity. Then try reducing that time by one, two, or three hours a day—it will be the easiest, least expensive health dividend you can invest in. You might want to use an app or notification software to remind you to get up and stretch, change position, or do some other type of movement.

If you sit at a desk much of the day, invest in one of the many standing or treadmill desks, most of which provide a flat space for laptops and tablets. Your hands and eyes can be busy while the rest of your body is moving. Most users report that far from being distracting, the movement increases their ability to concentrate as blood flows into the brain. Use extreme caution however. Falls on a treadmill can be lethal.

For phone calls, use a headset, walk around, swing your arms, and get up on your toes while you talk on the phone. Walk to colleague's offices rather than using the phone or text messages to communicate. If you want to write memos, dictate them into a device while you are stretching, walking, or climbing up and down stairs.

If you still watch old-fashioned TV, stand up and stretch when the commercials come on or even during the program. Set up an ironing board and do the ironing you never get around to.

3. *Movementize* **your life.**

Take the stairs instead of using the elevator. Have a walking meeting with a colleague after lunch and discuss an issue as you stroll around the block or to a local park. Tap your foot when you're sitting in traffic. Do chores.

Recently, I did a little experiment. What if instead of having all the phone numbers I needed on my mobile phone, I used an actual phone book to look up the numbers? I could keep it near the kitchen desk where we set the mail, because I'm often at the other end of the house, so that would force me to take a walk whenever I needed to find a number. In one day, I went back and forth three times. That was a few hundred steps just going for the phone book. Count out the steps in your daily routine and see where you could create routines that naturally add steps to your day.

Park your car at the far corner of the parking area and walk to your office building. If you often order in lunch, place your order for pickup, skip the tip, and be your own delivery person. If you have an electronic garage door, get out of the car to open the door anyway. That adds steps to your daily count, works your muscles, and contributes to your flexibility. Ride your bike to the nearby corner market when you need to pick up just one or two things.

Take vacations that include a lot a natural movement—plan for walks, hiking, golf, museum going, or swimming. You'll reset your sense of what makes for a healthy day, which will carry over into your daily life once you're back home.

4. **Get outdoors.**

Location, location, location. Although any exercise you do is good exercise, getting your movement outdoors in a natural area has extra benefits that working out inside doesn't offer. In a study of runners, it was found that the group that ran on a treadmill in a gym expended less energy than the group that ran outdoors and had to adjust for terrain changes and wind pressing against them. Running downhill as you often do outside flexes and engages different muscles than running uphill or on flat ground. Biking is another way of getting outdoors for exercise and working with the natural elements of wind and gravity to get extra benefit from your movements. Consider buying an e-bike. It takes the intimidation out of tackling monster hills, rekindling the romance of riding a bike outside.

More importantly, research shows that "green" exercise outdoors—where you are exposed to sunlight, plants, and natural settings—causes an increase in positive feelings. Simple walking in nature is one of the best things you can do for yourself. Greater enjoyment and satisfaction will make you want to repeat the activity—which explains why outdoor exercisers tend to stick with their routines more consistently than indoor exercisers do. Exposure to plants outdoors decreases levels of the stress hormone cortisol, too.

5. **Look for ways to include the four elements of exercise.**

To realize the full health benefits of movement, look for ways to incorporate the four elements of exercise into your daily and weekly routines, including training for strength, endurance, flexibility, and balance.

Strengthening (resistance) training. Strong muscles means we can lift objects and easily get up and down from a chair and ascend and descend flights of stairs. Being physically strong also creates an inner sense of confidence and capability. Strength, or resistance, training can include training with your own body weight, dumbbells, barbells, resistance bands, or weight machines two to three days a week, ideally using all the major muscle groups of the legs, abdomen, arms, chest, back, and shoulders.

Endurance (cardio or aerobic) training. Endurance fitness—including walking, jogging, dancing, tennis, and other active sports—means we can do all the things we want to from climbing stairs (and mountains) to protecting our hearts, and much more. The National Institutes of Health guidelines say that we should try to get 75 minutes of intensive aerobic activity or 150 minutes of moderate activity per week, but *almost any amount of walking or aerobic exercise will help protect and improve your heart and health.*

Flexibility (stretching) training. Stretching improves flexibility. Current thinking no longer recommends stretching before exercise but rather midway or afterward, when the body is already warmed up. Stretching activities that lengthen and stretch muscles can help you prevent injuries, address back pain, improve balance and posture, and basically increase your ability to use your whole body and range of movement. That's a wonderful feeling. There are many, many exercise videos available online to get you started. Just be careful! Make sure your muscles are already warmed up and don't push or force. Think Dr. Su's advice: "Happy energy, happy exertion."

Balance training. Balance training is critical to prevent falls, and the National Institutes of Heath says that people 65 and older should do balancing exercises to prevent falls—but why wait? People who sit a lot—at work, at home—can lose some of their sense of balance that they had earlier in life. If you're noticing any balancing problems, and even if you're not, you should make sure you're doing some balance training in midlife. Leg lifts (to the side and back and forth), the stork pose (balancing on one foot with arms held out to the side), yoga poses, and other exercises, such as heel-to-toe walking slowly, can help you develop greater balance and stability. One woman I know plays a video game her kids have that features several balancing games—she tries to beat her kids' scores. She also takes a weekly dance class that makes her turn her head and spin, and she stops to do yoga poses throughout the day. She says all three types of movement seem to have helped her regain balance that she had been losing gradually from sitting a lot.

> "FOR INSPIRATION, I LIKE TO REMIND MYSELF:
>
> TAKE CARE OF YOUR BODY. IT'S THE ONLY PLACE YOU HAVE TO LIVE."
>
> —Jim Rohn, entrepreneur

6. **Find a movement mate ... or two or three.**

One of the challenges that we are faced with is staying motivated to exercise. About half the people who join a gym don't stick with it beyond the first year. It can take a while to find the right companions who can help you get motivated to work out with them when you are in the mood to skip it, but having a walking or exercise class companion can make all the difference. One highly fit 70-year-old I know, a retired philosophy and French professor with a lifelong passion for languages, met a Russian émigré at his local Y and the two of them started a weekly Saturday morning walk. He'd get a Russian lesson on the two-mile walk along the beautiful path they took. On the return they'd switch to a French lesson.

7. **Just walk.**

Remember, just walking each day has the potential to reduce risk for disease, and it's something that most people are physically capable of doing with minimal risk for injury. Measure the steps you take daily and then find ways to double it. Just give it a try.

8. **Safety comes first.**

If you have any chronic health conditions, or have balance problems or any health issues that might limit your ability to exercise, be sure to consult your health care provider before you start an exercise program to find out about the types of activity that might be appropriate for you. Also, remember to drink plenty of water during physical activity. Older adults sometimes don't feel thirsty, even though they need fluids, and exercise will make you need to hydrate yourself.

Short on Time?

One of my friends swears by "The Scientific 7-Minute Workout," a form of high-interval intensity training that she read about in the New York Times: It's a series of 12 exercises, all gentle on the joints, that combines aerobic, balance, strength, and some flexibility movements, each done for 30 seconds with short breaks in between. My friend thinks of her seven-minute workout as part of her morning routine, like making the bed, and she'll add on a short jog or walk on most days. The original version and variations of the workout are on YouTube and there's even an Alexa app. Other variations of quick workouts include "high-intensity interval training" or "high-intensity intermittent training" workouts where you briefly do intense movement—like running in place as fast as you can—and then rest for a short interval before briefly going back to the intensive movement and repeating the sequence several times.

CHAPTER FOUR

Your Healthy Edge

DEVELOPING RITUALS OF DAILY MOVEMENT

Movement is crucial for keeping your body strong, flexible, and healthy throughout your life. The ideas listed below can help you ensure your body remains as vital as it can be throughout your life.

- ☐ Purchase a pedometer and track how many steps you take on an average day. Set a goal to double that number.

- ☐ Track how much you sit and how much you move for one week.

- ☐ Request walking meetings at work at least two to three times a week to improve your blood flow and productivity and increase your step count.

- ☐ Use a standing desk at work to avoid sitting too much.

- ☐ Walk 30 minutes after dinner four times a week to improve digestion and increase your weekly movement.

- ☐ Forest bathe once a week to get in some gentle steps and improve your immune system.

- ☐ Take up qigong and/or yoga to improve posture, flexibility, movement, and breathing.

- ☐ Find ways to keep your movement continuous for one hour a day while at home (get all the chores done before you sit down, do your own gardening, play with your kids outside, cook dinner, or have most of the dishes done before you sit down to eat).

CHAPTER FIVE

Bring Me a Dream

CLEAN YOUR BRAIN AND RESTORE YOUR BODY WITH QUALITY SLEEP

"Finish each day before you begin the next, and interpose a solid wall of sleep between the two."

—RALPH WALDO EMERSON, AMERICAN PHILOSOPHER AND POET

In my opinion, sleeping well is the most important health habit to develop. In this chapter you'll learn how I changed from going to bed with a "fire brain" to methodically winding down each night so I sleep deeply, and give my body and mind a chance to recover from my busy day. Read on to learn how I did this and to discover:

- Dirty brains are linked to diseases like Alzheimer's and Parkinson's diseases. Quality sleep acts like a washing machine to clean your brain each night and protect you from these diseases and a myriad of other health problems.

- Sleep requirements change as you age, and there are different kinds of sleep, deep sleep in particular, that you need each night so your body can recalibrate and renew.

- Trying to catch up on sleep does not provide the same health benefits as getting the correct amount of sleep and sleep quality each night.

- Napping a bit each day really is good for you.

- Sleep apnea is a real health danger, but you can effectively treat it.

- There are steps you can take to improve your sleep, including unplugging early in the evening, making your bedroom conducive to sleep, and treating sleep like the health manna it is.

- Incorporate transcendental meditation into your routine, which is a wonderful brain cleanser and healer.

My whole adult life, no matter how well I was eating or how much I exercised, this is what it used to be like for me:

Fire brain.

At night.

During the day I was full-on from morning to evening, though I was good about getting a physical workout most days. After 45 minutes on the treadmill I would be dog-tired and ready to collapse, except I had to get straight back to work.

However, when bedtime came, I was so excited about all the things that I was doing that after 17.5 hours of go-go-go, I didn't know how to give my brain a break. I couldn't turn it off. My brain was so fired up that even when I slept, I didn't sleep deeply. My brain was taking all my body's energy, even during sleep.

On a typical night, I would be lying down at 10:30 or so, watching a violent, action-packed movie or a TV show like *Dateline* or *20/20* that was about a murder. With my iPad on my lap, I'd be triple-tasking by answering e-mails and texting on my iPhone at the same time. Eventually I'd crash and my body would fall asleep from pure exhaustion, iPad on my lap, phone in my hand, TV blaring, lights blazing. I had many dreams that woke me up and disturbed my sleep. My body might be asleep, but my brain was on fire.

I woke up tired, my weight was going up even as I tried to diet, my blood pressure and fasting blood sugar levels were rising—even my cortisol levels were getting higher. My lack of sleep was actually interfering with my body's essential healing and cleansing processes, though I didn't know it at the time.

If the purpose of sleep is to knit the cares of the day (a nod to Macbeth) into something you can put away as a memory and to refresh and clear the mind, I was definitely doing something wrong. If I hoped to live a long and happy life, something, maybe everything, had to change.

CHAPTER FIVE

Who Needs Sleep?
The Matter of Dirty Brains, Stressed Hearts and Bodies, and Emotional Overwhelm

In our 20s and 30s, it was a badge of honor to say we pulled all-nighters or kept going on three or four hours a night. Being overbooked was the ideal for many of us and it was popular to think that sleep was a waste of time. When you were 25 you could live on five hours of sleep and you could rock and roll. Whatever the health impact of pushing your body's limits, you could still manage; you had reserves of healthy capacity in your heart, lungs, circulation, and most important, your brain. You had a surfeit of neuron and cell production. You burned off some cells and replenished them faster than you could use them—until you got to a certain age, around 30, when the balance tipped. After that, your body started using more cells than it could replenish.

All of us were hurting ourselves and perhaps, ever so slightly, shortening our lives, but we didn't know it. We hadn't heard experts like James Maas, PhD, formerly of Cornell University, say, "Good sleep is the best predictor of life span and quality of life." Sleeping well is that important to our health and the actual cellular functioning of our bodies.

> "NIGHTLY REST IS NOT JUST PERFUNCTORY AMID INCREASINGLY BUSY LIVES—IT'S ACTUALLY CRITICAL TO SURVIVAL. THERE ARE SIMPLE THINGS WE HAVE TO DO TO LIVE, LIKE EATING AND EXERCISING. SLEEP IS ONE OF THOSE THINGS."
>
> —Conrad Iber, MD, Medical Director, Fairview Sleep Program (Minneapolis)

Now it's time for a reckoning.

Lack of sleep is also making America less civil. Lawrence Epstein, MD, head of Harvard's Sleep Health Centers, backs this idea up in an article titled "Sleep and Mood," which states 35% of Americans don't get the recommended amount of sleep, which is making us cranky and a less civil nation. Add the widespread problem of metabolic syndrome to sleep deprivation, and civility, in my opinion, plummets even more.

Over the years, scientists have made amazing discoveries about what actually happens when we sleep. New techniques that peer into the brain show that sleep is essential for at least three distinct functions:

- Cleansing the brain of toxic buildup

- Storing memories

- Maintaining metabolic balance for neuron and cellular health

That's pretty powerful stuff. The results in terms of well-being are real: lack of sufficient or deep enough sleep leads to greater risk of brain and memory impairment, heart disease, insulin and hormone imbalances, and the emotional fallout of worry and anxiety when the mind can't or won't turn off.

The Washing Machine Metaphor: A New Understanding of Brain "Washing"

I tell everyone I meet: your brain needs sleep to detoxify. That's what the new brain imaging studies are showing us. Our bodies need to cleanse themselves. Our skin naturally sloughs off its top layer. Our digestive system rids our bodies of waste and toxins. (In addition, we can cleanse our intestines with fasting and other rituals.) The body uses the circulatory system for transporting blood and nutrients to where they need to go and uses the lymphatic system for clearing the body of wastes. However, it was believed for a long time that the brain was the only part of the body that didn't have its own built-in lymphatic system—just a circulatory one.

> IF YOU INTERRUPT YOUR SLEEP, YOU CAN'T WASH YOUR DIRTY BRAIN.

Neuroscientist Jeffrey Iliff, PhD, and his team at the University of Rochester Medical Center, discovered that the brain does have its own washing system, which they call the glymphatic system. It has a unique role in cleansing our brains—at night when we're asleep!

Each of our cells functions like a miniature factory, producing chemicals and fueling processes in our bodies. Like factories, and like all the cells in our bodies, our brain cells also produce waste that must be flushed out.

Dr. Iliff and his team discovered that the human brain has developed an ingenious system for ridding itself of waste. The clear cerebrospinal fluid (CSF), which is found between the cells in the brain, carries the waste along the outside of the blood vessels. But Dr. Iliff discovered that when the brains of mice go to sleep, their brain cells shrink and the space between them expands, allowing the fluid to rush through and clear out waste. During the day, the brain puts off this cleansing process. As Dr. Iliff explains, it's similar to how "we put off our household chores during the week when we don't have time to get to [them], and then we play catch-up on all the cleaning that we have to do when the weekend rolls around."

When you go to sleep at night, your brain flushes its dead cells out of your body. If you interrupt your sleep, you can't wash your dirty brain. When you lack sleep, two things are going on—both of them bad. The first is that your body is not allotted the time it needs to produce new cells. The second thing is even worse. The waste in the brain includes amyloid-beta, a protein that is continuously produced in the brain, which can build up and aggregate as plaque in the spaces between the brain's cells. If you're not sleeping well, you don't allow the full wash cycle to take place, so that sticky plaque clumps and clusters—and guess what happens? Though the science is not yet definitive, it likely results in memory loss, Alzheimer's disease, dementia, and other "dirty brain" diseases like Parkinson's, which are caused by, correlated to, or sped up by the lack of sleep.

Researchers at Johns Hopkins studied 70 older adults, average age 76, who were part of the ongoing Baltimore Longitudinal Study of Aging. Using brain scans, they found that the participants who said they got the least sleep, less than five hours a night, or who did not sleep well had higher levels of amyloid-beta in the brain than those who slept more than seven hours a night.

While the researchers couldn't say whether poor sleep caused the buildup or the buildup caused the poor sleep, or if both effects were true, the study's lead author, Adam Spira, PhD, explained, "These findings are important, in part because sleep disturbances can be treated in older people. To the degree that poor sleep promotes the development of Alzheimer's disease, treatments for poor sleep or efforts to maintain healthy sleep patterns may help prevent or slow the progression of Alzheimer's disease."

So, How Much Sleep Do We Really Need?

As we age, our sleep needs change. Newborns require 14 to 17 hours of sleep a day. Teenagers need eight to 10 hours and adults generally need seven to nine hours. Except for about 2% of the population (odds are, you aren't in that group), everybody absolutely needs at least seven hours of sleep a night. Sleeping less than six hours or more than nine hours is associated with increased health problems and mortality, so if either fits your sleep pattern, you might want to look into whether you are getting too little or too much sleep.

Sleep becomes ever more important as we age. In our late 30s, the deep, memory-strengthening and restorative stages of sleep start to decline. While the common belief that humans need less sleep as they age is a myth, older people do tend to sleep more lightly and for shorter durations. Thus we have to do everything we can to maximize our sleep in order to protect our minds, cell generation, and the peak functioning of our bodies.

Deep Sleep and REM: Timing Is Everything

Getting enough sleep is only part of the sleep issue. Getting the right kind of sleep is just as important. A full 20% or 25% of the energy our bodies generate supports the activities of our brains. When we get "good" sleep, that energy can be used to support and replenish all the systems in our bodies, including essential cell growth. It's a big *if*, however, because so many of us have trouble getting a good night's sleep, as my fire brain experience showed.

So what is "good" sleep?

Sleep patterns are described in terms of eye movement. REM, or rapid eye movement, sleep is the stage of sleep that involves dreaming. Non-REM sleep happens in four stages: (1) drifting in and out of light sleep; (2) slowing of brain waves and disengaging from surroundings; (3) extremely slow brain waves (delta waves), interspersed with smaller, faster waves; and (4) almost exclusively delta waves. Stages three and four are what experts consider deep sleep, which is the most restorative, "good" sleep we are aiming for. Track these stages with a sleep monitor. According to the National Sleep Foundation, you should be getting about 15% to 25% of REM sleep and 12% to 25% of deep sleep each night.

It's during deep sleep that our blood pressure drops and our breathing slows. The blood supply to muscles increases and tissue growth and repair happens. Hormones that regulate growth and appetite get released. The brain takes the stimulation, events, learning, and insights of the day, sorts them out and processes them to determine their larger meaning, and transfers them to places in the brain where they are stored long-term.

REM sleep alternates with the four stages of non-REM sleep. During REM sleep, our breathing is rapid and irregular, our eyes jerk rapidly, and our limbs become immobile and relaxed as the brain's usual signals to the muscles are turned off.

As the night wears on, our sleep cycles shift. Longer periods of deep sleep tend to occur in the early part of the night, before midnight, and longer periods of REM sleep happen toward daybreak. That's true regardless of when you go to bed. If you generally retire after midnight, even if you sleep eight hours, you may not be getting enough of the deep, restorative sleep you need for peak cognitive function and memory.

Sleep Debt:
Are You Suffering From Lack of Sleep?

The hours registered on your bedside clock only tell you how many hours you were in bed, not the actual quality or quantity of your deep sleep. These are the questions I ask my friends, my colleagues, and the families I meet at our communities when they "wake up" and start to worry about their sleep:

- Do you often wake up tired, with a bad headache, and have to drag yourself around during the day?

- Do you get up in the middle of the night disoriented and confused?

- Does your significant other complain about your snoring and gasping for breath during the night?

- Are you suddenly experiencing fatigue all day long, feelings of being out of breath, or other signs and symptoms of heart disease? (Don't delay seeing your doctor or going to the emergency room if you're experiencing pain.)

- Are you suffering from irritability, worry, anxiety, depression, recurring negative thoughts and ruminations you can't stop, or lack of motivation?

- Are you dealing with weight gain issues, diabetes or prediabetes, or food cravings and bingeing that could be triggered by the stress hormone cortisol (which sleep helps control)?

- Are you worried about being less productive and effective, scared about increasing "senior moments" and mental gaps like forgetfulness, poor concentration, poor decisions, or carelessness?

If you answered yes to any of these questions, you may need help developing your sleep habits for better health.

We know that every year, an estimated 40 million Americans suffer from a chronic sleep disorder. The most common ones are insomnia, where you have trouble falling or staying asleep (or both), and sleep apnea, a condition of compromised breathing, which results in diminished oxygen being supplied to your brain. (You'll learn more about that later.)

Not getting enough sleep weakens your immune system, raising the risk for infection and some types of cancer. Your body's ability to metabolize glucose decreases, causing insulin sensitivity, which makes you more vulnerable to diabetes. Without enough sleep, your body decreases its leptin and increases its ghrelin.

One study of more than 83,000 healthy American men and women in midlife (age 51 through 72) looked at their self-reported sleep and weight changes over an average of 7.5 years. The study, "A large prospective investigation of sleep duration, weight change, and obesity in the NIH-AARP diet and health study cohort," found that those who slept less than five hours a night had a 40% higher risk of becoming obese than those who slept seven to eight hours a night.

In addition to shortening your life, sleep deprivation is both dangerous and debilitating. It leads to slow reaction times, irritability, and inattention. The National Highway Traffic Safety Administration estimates that sleep-deprived drivers cause 1 million motor vehicle accidents and at least 1,500 fatal crashes per year.

If you do shift work or have a work schedule that challenges your ability to maintain a healthy sleep schedule—something that is becoming more common in our 24-7 kind of economy—you're at real risk for health problems and will need to work extra hard to get enough sleep. Some 22 million Americans are affected. This includes people working in traditional trades of law enforcement, health care, and manufacturing, retail, information technology, and media, as well as anyone who travels for business or has a long commute, requiring them to start their day early in the morning. Shift work in particular makes it extremely difficult to get enough consistent deep sleep and to have circadian rhythms that enhance health and peak performance.

Anxiety, depression, and worry are exquisitely connected to lack of sleep and to sleep disorders. A cycle of worry and negative thoughts can keep someone awake all night. Negative, obsessive thinking and a sense of not having control of your thoughts can feed on itself and soon you are worrying about worrying, reinforcing the rumination. People who get less sleep and go to bed very late often experience more negative thoughts than people who have more regular sleep cycles and get to bed earlier. Researchers Meredith Coles, PhD, and Jacob Nota, PhD, of Binghamton University of the State University of New York suggest that helping people get to sleep at the right time, much earlier in the night, could have a direct positive impact in preventing as well as improving episodes of depression and anxiety.

> [PEOPLE] WHO SLEPT LESS THAN FIVE HOURS A NIGHT HAD A 40% HIGHER RISK OF BECOMING OBESE THAN THOSE WHO SLEPT SEVEN TO EIGHT HOURS A NIGHT.

In fact, the United States military has found that lack of sleep is one of the factors behind incidents of soldiers who commit acts of violence against others or themselves.

To Nap, or Not to Nap

In Europe and Latin America, daytime naps are part of people's lives, but this is less true in the United States. Even so, a short, well-timed nap has been shown to improve mental performance, combat daytime sleepiness, and elevate mood. JFK ate lunch in bed each day so he could take a nap immediately afterward. Reagan, Edison, and Churchill are other famous nappers.

I think of napping like plugging in your phone for 15 minutes when the power charge is low. Many studies show that 10 to 20 minutes is optimal, though for some people a nap of 90 minutes or so works, which allows for one complete sleep cycle. Naps that fall in between produce sleep inertia and can make you confused and groggy, although the benefits may still occur once the postnap alertness returns.

Timing is important, too. Most benefits seem to come from taking a nap in the afternoon, when alertness dips, usually between 3 and 5 pm Taking a nap between 7 and 9 pm can result in prolonged sleep inertia and is likely to interfere with the ability to fall asleep later that night.

Napping can be an energy and clarity boost, but it's not a cure for poor sleep.

Don't kid yourself that you can easily make up for lost sleep. Yes, you might still be able to pull off an occasional all-nighter at 50, 60, or 70 to get you through a big deadline or marathon trip. But you know how long it takes to recover from jet lag. Imagine doing that to your body regularly.

Charles Czeisler, PhD, MD, FRCP, professor of Sleep Medicine at Harvard Medical School, insists, "You can't catch up on lost sleep," which he calls "sleep debt." If you occasionally miss a few hours of sleep during the week and catch up by sleeping in on the weekend, you have a low amount of sleep debt. You may be able to repay that debt with a few hours of extra sleep on Saturday morning, but you will also be shifting your circadian rhythm, making it difficult to fall asleep on Sunday night and causing stress on your body as it works harder to find its right sleep-wake cycle.

"If you consistently miss a few hours' sleep each night for days or weeks on end, the accumulated sleep debt is as harmful as skipping an entire night of sleep," Dr. Czeisler explains. "Not only will it be physically impossible to catch up on the missing sleep, some evidence suggests that you may actually be permanently damaging your brain or causing other health problems that reduce longevity." Rather than think about how much sleep we can do without, we need to think of sleep as a vital sign that tells us about our well-being.

There's one silver lining, which is the creative thinking that can occur when we're tired; our analytical minds are more relaxed and we are more apt to free associate. This creative plus doesn't outweigh the risks of missing sleep, but it can help us take advantage of our fatigue. I'm sure this is controversial, but stay with me. According to work done by cognitive psychologist Mareike Wieth, PhD, when you're exhausted, you have lower inhibitions and are more willing to consider alternative perspectives and solutions you might have otherwise disregarded. Plus, your brain is more likely to wander when you're tired—and it turns out all that lack of focus can be great for sparking creativity. "That random thought can combine with your main thought and come up with something creative," Wieth said in *The Atlantic* article, "When Fatigue Boosts Creativity."

If you find "losing" some time in the middle of the night leads to creative breakthroughs, this might make you feel less frustrated by your night waking, even as you're working to get more of that better-quality sleep your body needs.

Of course this research hasn't been done with midlife and older adults, where the risks of lack of sleep are real and profound. In fact, for the thriving elders in our Aegis communities, nearly all say they were always "good sleepers" and only began having trouble sleeping when their health started to decline. Troubled sleeping seems to be one of the proverbial canaries in the coal mine of weakening health.

Apnea: A Sleep Disorder

So let's get back to sleep apnea and heart disease. Poor sleep can be exhausting to your heart. Especially with sleep apnea and related sleep disorders, you think you're sleeping, but if you're not in deep, restorative sleep cycles for enough of the night, your body can't rest, and your gasps for air put stress on your heart.

More than 12 million Americans have sleep apnea, a type of disordered breathing characterized by the tightening of the throat muscles, which usually relax during sleep to keep the tongue from blocking the airway. If the muscles tense up, the airflow can stop, sometimes for 10 seconds or more. The body goes into distress as the person gasps for air in their sleep, and this can happen hundreds of times a night. Sleep apnea can lead to high blood pressure, heart disease, stroke, memory loss, obesity, and insulin resistance. If you're over 50 and you have a neck size of more than 17 inches, you are at especially high risk.

Sleep apnea isn't a sleep disorder, it's a health disorder, and you could be silently wearing down your health and well-being.

A Journey With Sleep Apnea

In a TEDMED article called "Examined Lives: A Firefighter Lives Dangerously—While Sleeping," firefighter Thomas Zotti wrote about his experience with sleep apnea. His wife had pointed out that he was snoring, but he thought nothing of it—even when his doctor asked if he had any reason to believe he might have sleep apnea. Zotti worked overnight shifts and ignored some signs of problems: waking up from sleep feeling claustrophobic, experiencing headaches, feeling so fatigued that he stopped working out in the mornings. With coffee fueling him through his long days, he was able to mostly ignore his tiredness.

Boy, could I relate to his story—because I was having many of the same symptoms and, like Zotti, not connecting the dots. My snoring sounded like I was gasping for breath, according to my wife, but as long as it wasn't interrupting her sleep, I wasn't concerned. Zotti said that before he got treated for sleep apnea, the amount of oxygen in his bloodstream was as low as 81%—very low compared with the near perfect score in the high 90s that most people have.

Using a CPAP (a continuous positive airway pressure) machine while sleeping, or other treatments, people with sleep apnea can get the oxygen they need and get back their vitality. Certain CPAP machines work with mouth guards now. Sleep dentists specialize in mouth appliances to treat sleep apnea, too.

So if you are experiencing fatigue and you know that you snore, pay attention. While being a snorer doesn't mean you have sleep apnea, and not every person with sleep apnea snores, it's an important sign, especially as we age. Even if we didn't snore when we were younger, many of us will begin to snore as our soft palate tissue gets even softer, blocking the air passage, which is one of the most common causes of snoring.

The connection between snoring and sleep apnea can be especially strong for people who are overweight or where sleep apnea runs in the family.

10 Steps for Better Sleep

1. **Put out the fire in your brain and go to bed with your mind clear.**

   The first huge lesson I needed to learn was that I had to let my brain have downtime.

   Think about what thoughts you put in your head before you go to sleep. A work (or imagined) crisis that someone e-mails you about at 11 pm that will get your mind churning? A tension-raising text message that adds drama to a family issue? A stimulating action movie or a crime show? Or a CNN report on the latest terrorist attacks? You fire your brain up by putting these kinds of thoughts in it right before you go to bed.

   When I started to unplug from all devices two hours before I went to bed and switched from watching disturbing video and reports on TV to listening to music or reading a book before turning in, my sleep experience immediately changed.

   Meditation helps, too, even for five or ten minutes—or a warm bath. In Asian countries, there are qigong clinics where people learn how to heal their bodies through meditative states, which can have similar effects to napping and can help train the mind to unwind and fall asleep.

   The goal is to lower the intensity of your brain activity. If you think of your mind like a 10-rung ladder, the tenth rung, the highest one, is when your brain is on fire. REM sleep is the most active time for your sleeping brain, so fire brain keeps you on a high rung when what you really want is to descend down to rung one or two—the state of deep sleep. If you go to bed with your mind clear, you have a much better chance of getting healthy, restorative, deep sleep.

2. Shut off TV and electronics—the "blue lights"—one to two hours before bedtime.

We've all heard this: bedrooms are for sleep and sexual activity, not for TV and electronics. Many, many studies are showing that lights from these devices can fool the brain into thinking it should be awake. Screens emit blue light, and the blue light spectrum suppresses melatonin, a natural hormone secreted by the pineal gland in the brain. You need melatonin to regulate the body's circadian rhythm, your internal clock that tells you when it's time to fall sleep or wake up.

A healthy, regular circadian cycle allows the body to turn off and get a good night's sleep. It's equally essential to our daytime functioning once we wake up. A consistent rhythm of being asleep and being awake helps us stay alert, think clearly, and manage our moods and emotions.

To turn our minds and bodies off at night, we need to reduce or eliminate melatonin-stopping blue light before bed. Conversely, our central nervous system thrives on the healthy, broad-spectrum daytime light that literally makes our lives sunnier by regulating our brain's neurotransmitters and improving our moods.

The best thing is to turn all your electronic lights off one or two hours before bedtime and leave cell phones, tablets, and computers outside the bedroom. Second best is to try things like dimming your devices' screens, or using orange-lens glasses and screens, and putting soft white bulbs in your lamps. There are also new software applications like f.lux for computers and Twilight for mobile phones, which uses a red filter that protects eyes from blue light and allows melatonin levels to rise. This way, if you're up late looking at a screen, your body's ability to manufacture melatonin isn't disrupted.

Another option is to go on a weekend camping trip and try sleeping under the stars. That's how you can really reset your mind and body.

3. No alcohol four hours before going to sleep.

While alcohol in sufficient quantities will put you to sleep, it can prevent deep sleep and inhibit REM sleep. Alcohol may also cause you to wake up in the middle of the night, when it has metabolized and wears off. While studies have shown that one glass of red wine in the evening may help you sleep, three glasses will interrupt it.

4. **Cut evening caffeine.**

    This may seem obvious because caffeine keeps you awake, but I'm not just talking about the big latte eight hours before you go to sleep. Eating chocolate at 9 pm is just as bad and may keep you up because it contains caffeine. Other sources besides coffee and chocolate include nonherbal teas, some soft drinks, and some pain relievers. Don't trust your perceptions. You might think you're one of those people who isn't bothered by caffeine and you're able to get to sleep and stay asleep no matter what. Sleep lab monitoring is telling us that just isn't so. Caffeine consumed a full six hours before bedtime is shown to have significant detrimental effects on sleep. Why risk having caffeine interfere with that deep sleep you need, even if it doesn't actually make you wake up and toss and turn? This is why everyone should avoid caffeine consumption after midday, including coffee, caffeinated sodas, and chocolate.

5. **No foods, especially sugar foods and drinks, in the two to three hours before bed.**

    If you take a big drink of orange juice at 9:30 pm, that's going to set you abuzz because your body will race into action to handle all that sugar. Eating any food late in the evening is very likely to throw off your metabolism, so close up the kitchen well before bedtime.

6. **No strenuous exercise.**

    If you're the guy (or woman) who says, "Yeah, I like to go to the gym or spin class about 9 pm and then be in bed by 10:30 or 11," sorry, but that schedule isn't a good idea. Though your workout in the evening may not be intense enough to counteract the sleep-improving benefits of exercise, if you have any sleep problems or a history of insomnia, experts recommend you avoid exercise at least a couple of hours before bed. If you like some movement as part of your evening routine, try walking after dinner, doing light chores, or stretching and doing some gentle yoga poses instead, as long as you don't push your heart rate above 100.

7. **Create a conducive, restful environment.**

    Keep your room cool, dark, and comfortable. Our bodies cool down when we sleep and a warm room (above 68 degrees) competes with that natural cooling process. For women, dealing with hot flashes can be a challenge. It's important to have light sheets, light sleepwear, cooling pillows, and discussions with a doctor if hot flashes disturb your sleep.

Most of the steps for getting a good night's sleep won't cost you anything, but this one will: to the extent you can afford it, spend enough money on your mattress, sheets, blankets, and pillows to be sure they help you sleep well at night. There's a reason people say they sleep so well in nice hotels. Many of the worries of daily life have been left at home—lists of to-dos, bills to pay, and family conflicts. The rooms are dark, calm, and usually quiet. The mattresses and bedding are stellar. Even as you are trying to manage your stress and shut down your brain before bedtime, having a comfortable bed that helps you sleep soundly can be a smart investment in your health.

Seriously consider spending as much as your budget allows on a good mattress, and spend the money on the sheets and pillows you love and that will keep you cool and comfortable. Think about how much time you spend in that bed, probably nine hours a day, and how tremendous the benefit to your body and your immune system will be.

No matter what, make sure your mattress is not more than 10 years old. Second, make sure your bed is not too soft or too hard for you to sleep comfortably. Don't be afraid to return a new mattress that isn't "just right" and never buy a mattress you can't return or exchange. Also, if you and your partner have different sleep needs, consider a two-person option. There are mattresses that allow you to adjust the hardness and even temperature on both sides of the mattress so neither partner has to be uncomfortable.

With bedding, different fabrics have different cooling and heat-trapping effects. Aim for 100% cotton, but avoid thread-count gimmicks. Higher counts aren't necessarily better, and there are other factors that affect quality as well. If you're a woman experiencing hot flashes and night sweats, you might want to try moisture-wicking sheets that are now available.

8. **Plan your sleep.**

To establish good sleep habits you need to figure out the right sleep-wake schedule for you. It may not sound fun or exciting to have a regular bedtime, but that's the ideal and you'll thank yourself for setting it. Try to go to bed at the same time every night and get up at the same time each morning. Your body wants to be trained to go to bed at a certain time. It will regularize your circadian rhythm and set its own clock: "Oh, it's time to go to bed." You'll sleep better, and when your whole body is in sync and regularized, your moods, alertness, and ability to focus may improve.

9. **Develop shared sleep habits with your bed partner, or at least avoid disrupting each other's sleep.**

My wife and I have this discussion a lot, because I have really made sleep sacred. You have to be either on the same page with your partner about going to bed at the same time and waking up at the same time or respect each other's rhythms. Rhythm is very, very important. If you married your spouse when you were 30 and now you are 50, your body has gone through changes and you have to adapt to them.

If you and your partner have habits and schedules that don't mesh, find ways to honor your partner—read in another room, avoid having lights on or just use a small yellow-spectrum book light when reading in bed, use sleep masks, and so on. Having a shared ritual and commitment to sleep will be good for your relationship and your well-being, adding much-needed intimacy, relaxation, and restoration to your life and your partner's.

10. **Track your sleep.**

Every night in bed, I use a wearable device that monitors my movements to track my sleep. A good night's sleep for me is over 7.5 hours with more than two hours of deep sleep and two hours of REM sleep. Many of us go to sleep thinking, "Oh, if I go to bed at 11 and get up at 7, I'll have gotten eight hours." Once you start tracking your sleep, you'll be shocked at how often you wake up throughout the night. You get up to go to the bathroom and think it took five minutes, but your body actually woke up a few minutes beforehand and went to sleep a few minutes afterward, so that may have been a 20-minute event. If you wake up to adjust the blankets you may lose a little more. Each disruption can interfere with your ability to get enough deep sleep.

Waking up isn't the problem per se, so don't fret and panic about insomnia just because you get up. For example, a recent study looked at sleep patterns of people today living in isolated, indigenous cultures. It found that many in those cultures naturally have two sleep cycles and are awake for one to two hours in the middle of the night. History shows our ancestors had those patterns of sleep, too.

The point is to be aware of the total amount of sleep, the timing of that sleep (are you getting to sleep before 11 pm?), the consistency of your sleep and thus your circadian rhythm, and the amount of deep sleep you're actually getting to renew your body.

There are ranges of affordable devices that can track your sleep patterns. Some you wear, some you place on the bed, and some you put on your nightstand. I would bet the technology gets better and better as people become more aware of the importance of sleep and look for tools that can help them.

The False Panacea: A Note About Sleeping Pills

Too many of us—nearly 9 million Americans according to a CDC report—are relying on prescription sleep medications to fix a problem most of us don't actually have. We just think we have it. Our dangerous zolpidem culture is masking the real issue. In fact, drugs like zolpidem are associated with short-term memory loss. Clifford Saper, chair of neurology at Beth Israel Deaconess Medical Center, is quoted in the *Boston Globe* as saying drugs like Ambien, in the drug class imidazopyridine, cause what's called an amnestic response. He says that while the drug is active, you are not laying down any long-term memories, and "it is like a blank period in your memory."

Once we believe in the importance of sleep and take the steps to calm our fire brains, most of us can get a good night's sleep. If we're not sleeping well, we don't want to mask the often overlooked vital sign of sleep and miss the heart disease, depression, burnout, or health conditions that are screaming at us to notice them.

Sleep medications have their place, and getting sleep—even if you have to use an aid—is essential to good health. But many sleep medications have negative side effects, from altered states of consciousness to headaches. They can lead to dependence requiring higher doses over time—and even to addiction. They can cause drowsiness that next day when doses are too high and can lead to very serious consequences if they're mixed with other drugs and alcohol. Some people can experience erratic behavior and memory loss. With all these potential side effects, it's important to think twice about reaching for a medication instead of working harder to make lifestyle changes to support better sleep.

I really believe eliminating bad habits around sleep and replacing them with good ones, as outlined above, will decrease the need for sleep medication and give you the gift of a good night's sleep.

Have You Considered
Medical Marijuana for Sleep?

On my journey, and in doing the research for this book, I've come to believe that our health habits always need to be part of our "prescriptions" to prevent and cure illness and conditions. It is the positive lifestyle changes that enhance our cellular health and well-being. But sometimes medications and supplements, when customized to our bodies and needs, can be valuable adjuncts. That's how I'm seeing the potential of medical marijuana and cannabidiol (CBD) for sleep as well as for anxiety and other conditions. This is a personal decision, and although there is not a lot of scientific evidence, it's something worth looking at.

CBD, a derivative of marijuana that lacks the psychoactive component in THC, is calming, mild, and available in capsules and liquid drops. While research findings are still preliminary, CBD shows enormous promise for treating a wide variety of conditions including sleeplessness. So far, there aren't reports of the kinds of side effects associated with the other sleep medications out there. With more than half of US states allowing medical marijuana and CBD, it is something to discuss with your doctor before you consider using it (as you would with any drug).

Sleep is an innate, natural state of being—if we can just allow our minds to relax and our bodies to unwind. If we can get into a natural pattern of sleep, we'll naturally wake up refreshed and ready for our day. The habits of health alone are likely to lead to a good night's sleep and a good night's sleep helps us with everything else, especially our ability to feel happy and engaged in a purposeful, meaningful life, as we'll see in the next chapters.

Your Healthy Edge

DEVELOPING YOUR SLEEP HABITS

Now you know how crucial quality sleep is for promoting good health! The ideas suggested below can help you improve your sleep duration and quality, and therefore, your overall health.

- [ ] Reorganize your day so you are less active at night (e.g., exercise in the morning, drop an unnecessary nightly chore off your list).

- [ ] Wake up and go to bed at the same time each day.

- [ ] Turn off the TV and screened devices two hours before bed.

- [ ] Track the quality and duration of your sleep along with behaviors during the day and evening that contribute to your sleep quality (e.g., 55 minutes REM, one hour and six minutes deep sleep, ate dinner at 6 pm, no snacks, no alcohol, meditated before bed, read a paper book).

- [ ] Make your bed and bedroom a haven for quality sleep (e.g., remove the TV from the room, invest in a quality mattress and bedding, hang blackout curtains so it's dark during the summer, or give yourself permission to nap).

- [ ] If you think you are a candidate for a CPAP machine, make an appointment with a sleep specialist to get a definitive diagnosis. After diagnosis, perhaps a sleep dentist can help you with an appliance that will improve your breathing, and reduce snoring, at night.

- [ ] Practice daily rituals to calm your overactive mind (e.g., mindfulness, meditation, deep breathing).

Hold Hands, Stick Together

CULTIVATE RELATIONSHIPS TO BOOST CONFIDENCE, HAPPINESS, AND HEALTH

"People who are most satisfied in their relationships at age 50 were the healthiest at age 80."

—Dr. Robert Waldinger,
DIRECTOR OF THE HARVARD STUDY OF ADULT DEVELOPMENT

Cultivating strong relationships is important for us all. I intentionally bring people into my circle of friends who I believe are kindred spirits, and I've also taken steps to release toxic relationships that drained me. In this chapter you'll learn that:

- Your health and longevity benefit from having deep connections with other people. These deep connections protect you from serious illness like dementia and Alzheimer's disease.

- A strong marriage is only part of the relationship equation. Friendships and strong social networks are even more important in terms of mortality rates.

- It's important to have friends who are 20 years younger than you. As you age, younger friends encourage you to keep up physically and spark your creativity.

- Happiness is the result of having great relationships, and happiness is what feeds optimism, health, and life satisfaction.

- There are some tried and true methods for developing relationships and feeding your happiness. Learning to listen and accepting yourself are among many listed in this chapter.

I sometimes wonder if friendship should be called "healthship." Social connections not only give us pleasure but also affect physical health. Many studies have demonstrated the health benefits of social connections—from a spouse or partner and extended family to best friends and loose but friendly ties. Feeling connected to other people can give you a sense of purpose and meaning as well as confidence that you can face challenges, learn new things, and be resilient. Having a strong social network lowers your risk of dementia, too.

There is a Harvard study that has followed more than 700 men since they were teenagers in 1938. These men came from all socioeconomic backgrounds; some had difficult lives, and others had it easier. The bottom line is that "Good, close relationships appear to buffer us from the problems of getting old," says Dr. Robert Waldinger, a psychiatrist and current director of the study. He also states that being in a securely attached relationship is protective in your 80s. Those people's memories stayed sharper.

One of the bright sparks of positivity at Aegis is a remarkable African American woman whose life mirrors the wrenching challenges of succeeding in segregated America. As a centenarian, her attitude is probably her greatest gift to herself and the wide circle of friends that have surrounded her for decades.

She was born in New Orleans in 1913 and worked as a helper in a pathologist's office starting when she was 11 or 12. In 1926, the doctor moved all the way to Seattle and he sent for her to come live with his family and continue working. She was only 13. The doctor helped her learn to read but she never went to school. As a teenager, she eventually moved to the YMCA and the housemother took her under her wing. The housemother introduced her to the black community and church, and she was taught etiquette and social skills with the other girls during their evening meals. She met her first (of three) husbands—a great example of the importance of a fulfilling life, not a "perfect" one. She had a vibrant community of friends. Apparently her phone never stopped ringing and she constantly had visitors and all kinds of committees and projects she was involved in.

When she thinks about what has been most important to her long life, she says:

> *I try very hard to be nice to people. I feel that down the road they too will be nice to everybody. I do things for someone, not because I want anything, but because I want the person to do the same thing—or more—for somebody else. The golden rule is one of the things I believe in. I feel it's paid off. Not everyone has done for me what I've done for them, but I feel like I've got it from somewhere.*

The Scientific Data on Relationships and Health

An analysis of 148 studies found that people with a network of friends and family that they feel emotionally connected to is extremely health protective. For example, quitting a smoking habit of 15 cigarettes a day or a drink habit of six drinks a day would not protect your health as much as having a circle of people who care about you. Of course, that's not an excuse to start smoking and drinking, but it's a reminder of how important it is to foster friendships and cherish the people around you.

I was surprised that the scientific data on the health benefits of relationships was so definitive and significant. We know we are social beings, but we're not taught to connect our friendships to our health. We need to. Our marriages are only a small part of the connection equation.

Yes, having a good marriage can contribute to a positive attitude and practical and emotional support. But many studies show that friendships can contribute even more to your well-being and health. The Australian Longitudinal Study of Ageing looked at people aged 70 and above to see if social networks of children, relatives, friends, and confidants enhanced health. They found that having more networks with friends and confidants was protective against mortality during the 10-year follow-up period, while social networks with children and relatives were not significant with respect to survival.

A study of nearly 3,000 nurses, Nurses' Health Study, found that women without close friends were four times as likely to die from the disease as women with 10 or more friends. The amount of contact with a friend wasn't associated with survival—just having the friends was protective.

While many friendship studies focus on women, some research shows that men can benefit from friendships, too. More than 700 middle-aged Swedish men were studied for six years, and whether they were married or not had no effect on their risk of having a heart attack, but having friends did.

John Cacioppo, the director at the University of Chicago Center for Cognitive and Social Neuroscience, and his colleagues studied 2,100 adults 55 years and older and found that people who experience perpetual loneliness are at a 14% greater risk of premature death than those who do not. In a subsequent study, Cacioppo found that loneliness appears to trigger the fight-or-flight stress signal, which raises cortisol levels and inflammation—which by now you know is part of a chain of events that can dramatically affect your health.

Knowing all this, you can pay attention to your own social network. Think about whether you need to make new friends and where you can start to find them. Look to your peers, but also consider making new friends who are older and younger than you are.

Make New Friends, and Rediscover the Ageless You

In the many interviews and conversations I've had with people over 80, one of the pieces of advice that has rung the most true to me has been this: *You have to have friends who are more than 20 years younger than you.*

When I asked why, the person said, "Most of our friends who would be our age have died. If we were to do this all over again, by the time we hit 50 or 60, we'd start making friends with people who were 30 or 40. Plus younger people keep you on your toes. You can't live in the past. They make you think about the present *and* the future."

The octogenarians tell me, "Younger friends get us excited about things we wouldn't normally get excited about. They stretch us physically, expecting us to keep up with them. They stretch our creativity and get us involved with things we wouldn't normally do."

If you don't know younger people, think about your friends' children and your kids and their friends. One woman I know had a long habit of getting together with her girlfriends in her 50s, and one day she realized that some of the daughters and sons had interesting contributions to the conversations. Instead of just catching up with old friends, she decided to get to know their adult children better.

Have Young Children in Your Life

One of the simplest ways to lift our mood is to spend time with young people, whether that's watching your neighbor's baby so she can make a quick run to the store, volunteering at your local elementary school, or taking a good book to read at your local playground on weekends. Simply observing play and laughter can give us a respite from our worries and improve our moods.

Look at what you do socially. If you do meet new people but they all have gray hair—whether those strands are artificially covered over or out in the open—think about ways to engage with younger people. You might invite some peers and your mentees to a happy hour, or you could participate more actively in a business or social organization. I believe it is very important to have friends who are at least 20 years younger than yourself.

Through my foundation, D-One, I've consciously made time to mentor a handful of younger people, making sure I call or invite them to lunch during the year to provide advice and to be a sounding board on everything from business and career decisions to financial planning to making connections that can help them with a cause, new venture, or health-related referral. My horizons get expanded and I come away inspired by their ideas and potential.

> SOME OF YOUR "OLD" FRIENDS CAN BECOME NEW AGAIN IF YOU SEEK OUT NEW EXPERIENCES AND CONVERSATIONS TOGETHER.

Recently, my wife and I went out socially with a couple that was decades younger than we are. We had so much fun learning about what they were interested in, talking, and laughing that we realized we had stayed out at a bar with these two until 2 am.

My wife said to me afterward, "I feel like I'm 25 again." Doing something different can energize you and make you feel younger than you are. Discovering what people in their 20s, 30s, and 40s are talking about and interested in can help you challenge yourself to take risks and try new activities.

Companionship can take many forms. If you can't find a book club, group for walking together to get exercise, or a yoga-on-the-beach group, start one. Get some friends to join and put up a flyer at a coffee house or set up an event on social media. See what types of gatherings are announced in local, free newspapers with calendars of events, and see what's happening at community centers.

Seeking out new friends will improve your sense of purpose—it's a project in and of itself—with all kinds of unexpected rewards. If some of your efforts don't pan out, at least one will, and you'll surprise and learn about yourself along the way. Some of your "old" friends can become new again if you seek out new experiences and conversations together.

Great Relationships
Infuse Your Life with Happiness

Ultimately I believe happiness is what many people want along with longevity; and happiness has been proven to be life extending.

Recently I had the chance to meet Linda Evans, the star of the 1980s television show *Dynasty*. I asked her how she stayed looking so beautiful in her older age and she said, "It's the experience of being around positive people."

Research is proving what we've known from experience and observation about the value of a positive outlook and finding reasons to be happy even when faced with challenges. For example:

- People who perceive aging as a positive experience are more likely to practice healthy behaviors.

- People who think they're in poor health may die sooner than those who consider themselves healthy (regardless of their actual health status).

- Optimism, hope, life satisfaction, and happiness are associated with lowered likelihood of heart disease and stroke.

Furthering this idea about health and happiness, researcher, psychologist, and epidemiologist Andrew Steptoe, DSc, DPhil, at University College London, led a team that studied 30,000 people older than 60 for eight years to learn more about aging, health, and happiness. The study found that those who were least happy were 80% more likely to develop problems with everyday activities like dressing than the happier participants.

Dr. Steptoe and his team also analyzed the results of the English Longitudinal Study of Aging, which followed 11,000 people over 50. People who reported negative emotions like feeling anxious or worried were twice as likely to die within five years as people who reported feeling contented and excited. Steptoe has pointed out that this holds true regardless of age, economic status, or health status. Being happy despite challenges is health protective.

How to Improve Your Relationships, Happiness, and Mental Health

To enhance happiness and alleviate stress, depression, and anxiety, consider the following:

- **Let happiness be a guide.** Worry less about perfection and doing everything "right." If you follow all the "rules" of health but miss out on joy, pleasure, and a sense of purpose, you'll miss out on the health benefits of happiness.

- **Purchase experiences, not things.** Research has shown that purchasing things like new clothes and electronics won't make you happier overall. But buying experiences, such as travel or tickets to a play will maximize happiness. Anticipating the event and planning for it can provide even more enjoyment.

- **Try joining a group and be open to friends from new, different, or unlikely sources.** Read the flyers at the health food store and the library to find out what's happening in your community. Is there a gardening club or a bridge game advertised? A lecture where you might meet people interested in the same topic you want to learn more about? Take a class at a community center, church, or local college or university. You might want to think about lecturing, teaching, or leading a workshop if you have expertise you would like to share. Or volunteer to work for a cause.

- **Fake it till you feel it.** Research has shown that when you're feeling down, the mere act of smiling can cheer you up. Laughter can also slow your heart rate and reduce stress. Rent a funny movie or read a humorous book to improve your mood.

- **Join a laughter club.** Laughter is a tonic for health. Studies have shown that laughter can reduce stress, improve immune function, and even relieve pain. A number of laughter clubs have developed, where people gather to laugh and do breathing exercises. Find one at laughteryoga.org.

- **Practice meditation.** Meditation reduces stress, improves your mood, decreases your heart rate, respiratory rate, and blood pressure, and increases your production of serotonin and HDL numbers. Meditation can help you sleep better and maintain a better mood, reducing anxiety and depression. It also can help you be more focused and creative. Considering all it can do for our brains, minds, and bodies, we should all be looking at ways to meditate more. If you think you don't have time to meditate, consider this: a recent study has shown that the brains of longtime meditators were less affected by aging than the brains of nonmeditators. Maybe spending those extra minutes meditating will produce a longer, happier, and healthier life. Since meditation is associated with longer telomeres, it sure looks like time meditating is time wisely invested.

- **Practice mindfulness.** Mindfulness is a conscious attempt to pay attention to the present moment in a particular way and in a nonjudgmental state. There's increasing scientific evidence that mindfulness can reduce stress, boost the immune response, improve sleep quality, and lower blood pressure and cortisol levels. You can sit to do mindfulness meditation or do mindful listening, eating, or walking. Search the Internet for instructions on how to practice mindfulness. You don't have to shut down all your thoughts and never let yourself get distracted. You just have to practice refocusing your attention on whatever you choose—your breath, or the feel of your feet on the ground as you walk very slowly.

- **Try yoga.** Practitioners of yoga, the ancient Indian health care practice, use breathing exercises, posture, stretching, and meditation to balance the body's energy centers. Yoga can reduce stress and anxiety and improve physical fitness, balance, and overall functioning. I talked about qigong and tai chi earlier. Yoga, too, should be seen as a gently flowing form of movement you can practice anywhere that will build strength, flexibility, and mindfulness.

- **Become a healthy habits master.** Getting enough sleep and physical activity, eating right, understanding your body, and being proactive about getting the care you need can all help alleviate stress and build your resilience.

- **Get specific help from a doctor or counselor if you're struggling with stress and moods.** There are treatments and medications that can alleviate depression and anxiety. If you're having a rough time managing your symptoms, talk to your doctor. Cognitive behavioral therapy is highly effective for the treatment of anxiety. It's shown to help people examine how their thoughts promote or worsen anxiety and how they can change them.

- **Join or start an exercise club.** Group activities will not only provide social support, but also promote healthy habits! For example, join a weight loss or walking club, or find a friend to walk with on a regular basis. Swimming or biking with others can get you out into the community and even into nature, depending on the climate you live in.

The Laughing Buddha Master

T and I were in India a while back. She wanted to try this yoga class across the street from the hotel at the Gateway of India. I agreed to go, but what I didn't realize was it started at 5 am. So I wasn't too excited about that, or the idea of the class, but I went anyway.

The class began with only one or two other people, and I'm thinking, "What am I doing here?" This very old, slightly built yogi leading the class says to us in broken English, "I want you to laugh like Santa … HO HO HO HO." We'd do a yoga pose to match. Then we laughed like a child: "HEE HEE HEE HEE," with a yoga pose to match. At this point I looked around and saw that a few more people had joined us. A few laughs later, even more people came. By 5:30, about 30 people were there and we were in hysterics. I could feel the blood flowing in my body and my mood was wonderful. By 6 am, people were there in suits before work, getting in a good mood and oxygenating their bodies before they began their day.

What we were experiencing was a community built around laughter and they used it to start their day in a very healthy way. The yogi, who has led the class for decades, is proof positive of the health benefits. He's 95 years old and offers this class five days a week as community service.

By the way, at the end of the class, with about 200 people now in attendance, I looked over at T and said, "I told you this would be great!"

A Friendship Refresher

If you feel your social skills are rusty or could use an upgrade, here are some ideas and tips:

- **Practice the art of socializing.** All skills take practice to keep them honed, and socializing is no different. Invite someone new for coffee or a walk. Not every opening will lead to a friendship, but you'll discover how happy it makes people to be asked. So reach out to new people and also old friends. As the saying goes, the phone works in both directions. Just because they haven't gotten in contact to plan some time for socializing doesn't mean they don't want to get together. Take the initiative, and when someone reaches out to you, accept the invitation.

- **Be a good listener.** Ask what's going on in their lives, and pay attention to what they say. When they share details of hard times, be empathetic but don't give advice, unless they ask for it.

- **Accept yourself and be positive.** Insecurity and self-criticism can be draining for friends on an ongoing basis and can turn people off to starting a friendship with you. Nonstop complaining can strain a friendship. Don't give an organ recital when asked how you're doing—"I'm having some stomach problems/heart trouble/lung issues." Share strategies for healthy living that you learned recently, but keep the focus on other topics: movies, what's happening in your community, or a book or article you read recently. Younger people don't gravitate toward older people because they have the feeling they're always talking about health issues, and our peers can get tired of comparing medical notes, too.

- **Accept others.** Don't judge. Become a little curious. Saying, "well, that's an interesting opinion" and asking questions to learn more can open people up and broaden your understanding of a variety of topics. People's stories about how they came to have a particular opinion or make a certain decision can be interesting. If your friends drive you crazy sometimes, remind yourself of what you enjoy about them. Give your friends space to grow and make mistakes even when you don't agree with their decisions. Encourage them to freely express their emotions without belittling them. If it's hard for you to deal with their emotions sometimes, remind them of their strengths, and tell them you have confidence in them. That can shift them away from telling you their woes and expressing their frustration over what you might think are minor problems.

- **Celebrate their good fortune.** Even if things aren't going well for you, friendship isn't a competition. Admire your friend's accomplishments and successes. Let them inspire you to believe that you can take on new challenges. If you envy their qualities and think you don't have them, start thinking about ways you might develop them. Get curious and creative and have some faith in yourself. You are never too old to make new discoveries about yourself, develop your talents, or try new activities.

- **Respect boundaries.** Try not to ask questions that may be too personal or make your friends uncomfortable. If you sense the other person is growing defensive or irritated, look for common ground and something to agree on. Later, you can acknowledge that you may not always agree, but you value your friendship and ability to be different from each other. Don't be too married to being "right." It's more important to be connected in friendship.

- **Be discreet.** Keep confidential any personal information that your friends share with you.

- **Express gratitude for their support.** Let other people you care about know that you appreciate them being there for you, and return the favor any time they're in need. Send a thank-you note, saying, "Gee, it's always so much fun to talk to you and hear what's going on in your life." A little gratitude goes a long way to nourishing friendships.

- **Rediscover or recommit to your religious or spiritual beliefs.** Some studies show church attendance and praying contribute to health and well-being. Being a part of a caring community that offers you a sense of purpose and focuses on the meaning of life rather than just the burdens of it can understandably help you develop happiness in your life. Prayer, like meditation and yoga, can for many people turn on the relaxation response of the nervous system, lower heart rate and blood pressure, and cause deeper breathing. In fact recently I was talking to a nun and learned of the 72 members in her convent: 35 were over 90 with the oldest being 106! So in the name of longevity, be open to exploring your spiritual nature and taking up spiritual or religious practices to discover whether they have meaning for you. They may help you feel you are part of something larger than yourself that is meaningful and positive. It's never too late to develop your spirituality.

- **Remove toxic friends from your life.** Don't let history decide who your friends should be. Don't have friends for their status, money, or fame if you really don't like being around them. Have friends with positive energy and who make you feel good about yourself.

Pets: Our Furry Friends

Even if you're not married or don't have a large social network, you may be able to get help from a furry friend—or a feathered one.

"The general belief is that there are health benefits to owning pets, both in terms of psychological growth and development, as well as physical health benefits," says Dr. James Griffin, a scientist at NIH's Eunice Kennedy Shriver National Institute of Child Health and Human Development. Though there have been relatively few well-controlled studies, we do know that time with pets can lower blood pressure and help us return to a calm state after stress. Dog owners also get regular exercise walking their pets and have opportunities to socialize with others as they meet other dog owners or talk to people on the street or at a dog park.

You might think having a dog is a lot of responsibility, but think about how a dog might contribute to your health. Cats and other furry companions might be good for your health, too, simply by being there for you to enjoy taking care of and petting.

Your Healthy Edge

DEVELOPING RELATIONSHIPS

Deep relationships with people other than your spouse or partner are shown to elevate a person's well-being because people with deep relationships are much more satisfied and happy than those who are lonely. Try a few of these ideas on for size and see if they help you strengthen existing relationships or make new ones.

- ☐ Set a date with each of your closest friends to see a play, hear a lecture, or go out to a new restaurant (ideally something that the two of you have never done together that would be memorable).

- ☐ Expand your circle of close friends by asking a person you admire, but haven't spent much time with, to coffee and learn if a deeper friendship might be formed.

- ☐ Purchase experiences with your friends rather than buying them material things (e.g., vacationing for a weekend, going to the theater or a museum, or taking flying lessons together).

- ☐ Join a local laughter club to make friends and improve your health at the same time.

- ☐ Become a better friend by becoming a better listener.

- ☐ Adopt a pet to learn how to give love and receive it unconditionally.

- ☐ Become good friends with at least one person 20 years younger than you (e.g., your kid's friends, your hairstylist) or become a mentor or a coach at a local school.)

- ☐ Rid yourself of toxic relationships (e.g., friend, boss, coworker, spouse, and family members).

My Reason for Being

NURTURE YOUR PURPOSE AND FEED
YOUR OPTIMISM TO FIND HAPPINESS

"Happiness cannot be pursued; it must ensue.
One must have a reason to 'be happy.'"

—VIKTOR FRANKL,
AUSTRIAN NEUROLOGIST, PSYCHIATRIST, AND HOLOCAUST SURVIVOR

Purpose is paramount in my life, and I think that's just the way I'm built. But what I didn't really understand before writing this book was that my purpose brings me such happiness, gratitude, and optimism for the future. Your purpose can bring the same health-giving energy to your life as well.

In this chapter I further explain that:

- Having a reason to wake up in the morning because you are needed helps improve your health and extend your life.

- Setting goals and pushing yourself increases your likelihood of thriving in your later years.

- Positivity is an excellent health tonic. Plus, cultivating resilience and optimism can feed your sense of purpose and vice versa.

- Happiness is fed by your sense of purpose, and Dr. Su also offers other ways to improve your happiness, like giving yourself permission to be happy.

- If you see aging in a positive light, you are more likely to practice healthy habits.

One of the most significant books I've ever read is Viktor Frankl's *Man's Search for Meaning*. To this day, his life and work inspire me. A prominent neurologist, psychiatrist and Holocaust survivor, he worked as a therapist in the concentration camps. Seared in his experience was this insight:

Everything can be taken from a man but one thing, the last of freedoms—to choose one's attitude in any given set of circumstances, to choose one's own way.

Frankl found that those who survived believed there was something expected of them in the future—they had some purpose to fulfill. He famously said, "It is characteristic of the American culture that, again and again, one is commanded and ordered to 'be happy.' But happiness cannot be pursued; it must ensue. One must have a reason to 'be happy.'"

That's what I've seen and believe. While we can't control our life circumstances, we can do our best to find ways to promote happiness, purpose, and well-being. The physical, emotional, intellectual, and spiritual elements of life all promote our healthy longevity. Living in a state of suffering, anger, or anxiety, on the other hand, leads to the opposite of health, just like too much sitting or not enough sleeping.

As you read about some of the research on longevity and happiness, you might start to think, "That's something my grandmother told me once." Studies show she was right about quite a lot when it comes to a positive outlook and not letting yourself get too wound up about the things you can't change. Even so, you might be surprised by some of the discoveries researchers are making.

Let It Go

Don't ignore the value of letting go of what isn't working for you, whether it's a too-stressful job or a relationship or something else, like a habit of letting people push your buttons. It is never too late to reinvent yourself.

There is no law that says midlife and older people don't and can't change. All the research on aging shows that people do continue to evolve and grow throughout their lives. Undertreated anxiety or depression at any age is not necessary. There are solutions and you can harness your resilience and feel optimistic about your future.

The Purpose Effect

To some, purpose means having a sense of direction and overarching goals, or even specific ones—like learning a language or how to play the piano or guitar. What I've come to understand is that no matter what a person's purpose, it can be defined as a reason to wake up in the morning because you're needed—by an endeavor, a spouse, a community, or grandchildren.

A sense of purpose organizes your time, focus, and even relationships. If you have to get out of bed to start making phone calls and organizing for a community event you are involved in, it's easier to push yourself out of bed and get moving.

I understand purpose as putting forth effort toward doing things that have meaning for you and having daily, doable microgoals. You're the one who decides what gives you purpose. Look at gardening as just one example. If gardening has become a passion for you, giving it a sense of purpose in your life would lead you to read gardening books, talk to neighbors about what they're planting and share ideas and tips, speak to experts at nurseries, and move things around in your yard to improve and enhance their health and visual impact. You get the idea.

Dabbling—putting forth minimal effort instead of pushing yourself to learn more, create more, and contribute more—doesn't give rise to satisfaction and doesn't grow a sense of purpose. Being able to give someone advice on where to plant a particular flower or bush on their lawn or helping your gardening club put on a plant sale can make you feel connected to others around you. Learning about something new from others can do that, too. Think about what you can share with other people and what you can learn that will make you feel energetic.

Renewed Sense of Purpose

People who have goals and work toward them are likely to feel a sense of self worth and fulfillment, which helps them maintain a positive outlook on life. While research shows that finding purpose early in life is a prescription for health, I believe that finding a *renewed* sense of purpose is what takes people into thriving later in life. If you are bored with gardening after many years of doing it, find a new way to garden—or a completely new hobby or pursuit that excites you. If you live to 100 or beyond, you will have several lifetimes of purpose and passions to fulfill.

Hidekichi Miyazaki, a Japanese father of four and grandfather of 10, was 105 years old in 2015 when he completed the 100-meter sprint in 42.22 seconds and set a new Guinness world record in track and field as the oldest competitive sprinter. He also competed in the shot put event at the Kyoto Masters Tournament.

What struck me most about his life wasn't his competitive running or his race times. It was his sense of purpose. Before he took up track and field at the ripe age of 93, he spent 33 years practicing calligraphy and playing Japanese chess with his friends. Those habits gave him purpose and friendship for many years. But as his friends started to die from old age, he wanted to find something he could do on his own—thus the track and field events.

Miyazaki is vigilant about his training. According to his daughter, he practices every day, except when it's raining, in a nearby park. His routine is to run one 100-meter sprint and to practice throwing the shot put three times.

He refuses to "take it easy" and he has set a new goal to reduce his 42.22-second sprint time down to 36 or even 35 seconds.

His story shows that finding that purpose and happiness requires a bit of physical or mental effort—a stretching of the mind and body.

> I'VE COME TO BELIEVE THAT PURPOSE IS ABOUT GOAL SETTING AND HAVING A CONCRETE REASON TO GET UP EVERY MORNING. SPECIFIC, PURPOSEFUL GOALS PULL YOU INTO THE FUTURE.

I've come to believe that purpose is about goal setting and having a concrete reason to get up every morning. I've been investigating the goals that have shaped the lives of people over 80. Specific, purposeful goals pull you into the future, and like Miyazaki, many ordinary people do the extraordinary. Why not set high goals and enjoy working toward them?

One grandfather started a blog when he was 100 years old. Every day was an occasion to capture his thoughts and master the technology.

My friend's grandmother had worked for the Literary Guild Book Club for years after her husband died and eventually found a series of literary projects that were profoundly meaningful for her. In her late 60s she trained to teach illiterate adults to read. Meeting that goal required a long-term commitment to several students and tutoring sessions several days a week. In her mid-70s she came up with the idea of a library cart for a hospital that she could walk to from her apartment in

New York City. Three days a week she'd take the cart around a floor of the hospital and help people choose books. The conversations were as entertaining and healing to her and the patients as the books. In her 80s she read the Torah at a women's club at the local synagogue.

One elderly grandfather found meaning in playing tournament-level bridge with the goal of becoming a life master—and improving beyond that initial goal. He looked forward to finding new partners to play with who would challenge him to learn new strategies for winning. Improving his game was one of his passions.

> THE FACT THAT WE ALL DIE SOMEDAY SHOULDN'T BE AN EXCUSE OR A HINDRANCE TO HAVING GOALS.

Goals, learning, and connecting with new people can all contribute to a sense of purpose and keep you feeling excited about an activity.

Although we say that being in the White House ages United States presidents prematurely—think about all the jokes about President Obama's gray hair—research shows this isn't true. A 2011 study by S. Jay Olshansky, PhD, at the University of Illinois at Chicago showed that United States presidents of the last 50 years have lived, on average, eight and a half to nine years longer than the average American. These men held what's often called the most stressful job in the world—and we know high levels of stress can lead to an earlier death. Why, then, do so many presidents live so long after serving in office?

Maybe what these men have in common is that their lives were driven by purpose, and they were rewarded and praised for their hard work. Also, they carried over their purpose filled drive for meaning, and for making a difference after they served in office.

Jimmy Carter became involved in Habitat for Humanity, helping build houses for low-income people, and was an international peacemaker for decades. Bill Clinton developed a global foundation to connect and fund people with good ideas to solve problems like the AIDS crisis. He and George H. W. Bush worked together to help victims of Hurricane Katrina and the 2004 South Asian tsunami. George W. Bush quietly became an accomplished artist and published a highly praised book, *Portraits of Courage,* with his compelling paintings and stories of veterans. The project exemplifies the role of purpose.

Searching for a postpresidency pastime, Bush took up the unlikely activity of oil painting. His wife doubted he had any talent or could apply himself, but little by little, one day at a time, he worked with teachers, improved his skills, and executed an early work. Then, on the advice of a mentor, he applied himself to a subject dear to his heart—the wounded warriors of America's wars. Bush recalls playfully informing his first instructor: "Gail, there's a Rembrandt trapped in this body. Your job is to liberate him."

There wasn't a Rembrandt, but there was a Bush who dug deep, stuck with a long-term project, and created powerful, unvarnished close-up portraits paired with the narratives of veterans' personal experiences. The work captures an American story for all of us to witness.

The irony is, with the exception of Walter Mondale, United States Vice Presidents typically have not lived past age 76, the average mortality rate for men in the United States. I believe this is in part because they had a great deal of stress in their lives, but very little of the purpose, praise or rewards that comes with the presidency. After their term was over, they generally also did not develop a cause, mission, or purpose to carry them through the rest of their lives. If you think of what I'm saying as an equation–stress + no praise + no reward + no purpose = early death–¬you can see why you should take measures to turn that equation around.

We all have stress in our lives and this example illustrates why I strongly encourage you to live your life with positive purpose that brings meaningful rewards to you.

Purpose is Powered By Resilience and Optimism

To me, resilience—the ability to adapt positively to adversity—has always seemed to be a hallmark of longevity. I think that's one of the qualities that led to my interest in aging when I was just starting my career in my 20s.

I always remembered the time I was a young boy and met a World War I veteran in the home for the aging where my grandmother lived. On one of our weekly visits, I wandered the hall and heard a man calling for help. I tentatively walked into his room and retrieved his pillow that had dropped to the floor when my eyes saw all his medals. We started talking and I was spellbound by his war stories but also the stories of his productive—and now I see resilient—life.

The next time I visited my grandmother I went to look for him and found out he had died. I never forgot him and when I got my first job working with the elderly, the thing that made the work meaningful for me was spending time talking to the residents.

Resilience and grit are being recognized as underlying keys to successful learning in young children—they lead to innovative thinking, perseverance, and delayed rewards. These are all things that help children experience the intrinsic rewards of learning. The same applies across the life span.

One Aegis Living resident comes to mind. He is 102 and hasn't had an easy life by any means—he became a refugee in World War II and lost everything. Yet he is cheerful, grateful, and resilient in the face of all the challenges he's faced. As he explains:

> *My health was bad and I was all alone during the war. I got sick and then we went to the relocation camp, a temporary one, and there were doctors but no medicine. When the war ended I had to start a new life.*
>
> *My life with my wife was the best thing for me. She turned me around. Mentally, she made me happier because I was in the doldrums all the time. She lifted me up. She did a wonderful thing. I can't get over it. She helped with my diet and everything. She understood. She fixed the food so I wouldn't have trouble. She knew all about me, more than I do about myself. I did my best to make sure that she was happy, too. We had no trouble. Since I was pretty active, we managed to have a pretty good life. Of course losing my wife ten years ago was the worst part, but the rest of it is all good memories.*
>
> *With the children, I managed to make enough to travel during vacation times. The kids still remember the old days—all the fishing trips, and the Grand Canyon, they remember everything. I'm thankful for that. I thought they'd forget, but they remember all of them. They don't remember the part when they got scolded.*
>
> *That's what keeps me going, the good memories.*

If you struggle to be optimistic and focus on the positive, there's some good news. Nir Barzilai, MD, director of the Institute for Aging Research at the Albert Einstein College of Medicine, says there is evidence that people can change their attitudes and behavior even at older ages. A study of 243 centenarians led Dr. Barzilai to discover that when it comes to personality, "we found qualities that clearly reflect a positive attitude towards life. Most were outgoing, optimistic, and easygoing. They considered laughter an important part of life and had a large social network. They expressed emotions openly rather than bottling them up."

> YOU MAY NOT KNOW RIGHT AWAY WHAT YOU CAN DO TO CHANGE YOUR SITUATION OR FEELINGS FOR THE BETTER, BUT BELIEVING THAT OPPORTUNITIES WILL SHOW UP KEEPS YOU OPTIMISTIC AND RESILIENT. THAT ATTITUDE CAUSES A CHAIN REACTION OF POSITIVE OUTCOMES.

Altogether, optimistic patients, and by extension, optimistic people, are more likely to do things to take care of themselves, including finding purpose in their later years. They believe they can make a choice that will lead to a better situation—and they don't have what psychologist Martin Seligman calls "learned helplessness," which is associated with pessimism. You may not know right away what you can do to change your situation or feelings for the better, but believing that opportunities will show up keeps you optimistic and resilient. That attitude causes a chain reaction of positive outcomes.

Purpose Can Improve Mental Health

I believe that having a strong sense of purpose does a great deal to lift one's mood and outlook on life no matter what a person's age. I also believe it's vital for improving mental health. Health researchers have known for quite a while that people with severe mental illness in general have shorter life spans, but they are starting to learn that milder conditions such as depression and chronic anxiety also have a very real impact on people's lives. Even low-level signs of depression and anxiety may be associated with a 20% increase in health risks. Chronic stress can lead to a string of problems, including increased cortisol and inflammation, a depressed immune system, metabolic changes, negative changes in the gut microbiome, brain disorders, and shortened telomeres.

My point is that to avoid this, especially as we age, make an effort to keep your sense of purpose alive and well. Being stoic instead of flexible and resilient, living in the past, and living without purpose and a sense of happiness are not the components of a prescription for health and wellness. There are so many options to improve your emotions and health. All the habits in this book have a direct connection to emotional well-being, but for anyone dealing with chronic unhappiness, rumination, anxiety, or worry, finding a sense of purpose and having healthy sleep practices are probably the first ones to adopt.

A note about depression: If you think you suffer from depression, something as basic as treating a hormone or vitamin deficiency may be in order. Testing can help you figure out if simply adding a nutritional supplement or changing what you eat could make a big difference in your mood. If you are suffering from depression, using an antidepressant medication may be an option, too. In addition, we know that meditation and exercise both can make you feel less anxious or depressed and help you relieve stress.

Shared Purpose Is Part of a Country's Happiness and Life Expectancy

According to the 2017 United Nations World Happiness Report, Norway and other Nordic countries top the list as the world's happiest nations. They achieved this in part through shared purpose. The report also notes that corruption in business and government are low in Norway, which in turn dials up the happiness effect for Norwegians, too.

The following excerpt is from the report's summary that links the country's economic and social success to shared purpose. "By choosing to produce its oil slowly, and investing the proceeds for the future rather than spending them in the present, Norway has insulated itself from the boom and bust cycle of many other resource-rich economies. To do this successfully requires high levels of mutual trust, shared purpose, generosity and good governance, all factors that help to keep Norway and other top countries where they are in the happiness rankings."

The report states that the other countries in the top 10 also have high values in all six of the key variables used to explain happiness differences among countries and through time—income, healthy life expectancy, having someone to count on in times of trouble, generosity, freedom, and trust.

Happiness in the United States Falls Dramatically

In 2007, the United States ranked third in the report. It fell to 19th in 2017 primarily due to declining social support and increased corruption. As an American, reading the report findings is quite unsettling. Income has increased a lot for just a few, and happiness is falling despite the "money is everything" drumbeat we all know well. The report's statistical analysis supports the idea that the United States could raise its happiness ranking by addressing its multifaceted social crisis due to "rising inequality, corruption, isolation, and distrust—rather than focusing exclusively or even mainly on economic growth, especially since the concrete [government] proposals along these lines would exacerbate rather than ameliorate the deepening social crisis."

To me this demonstrates the importance as an American to really begin working to create your own happiness through your strong sense of purpose. With a nod to Norway's success, developing a shared sense of purpose with others—in your neighborhood, at your kid's school, or at work—could go a long way to healing our country and our individual lives.

Beacons of Happiness

By now you're getting the idea that I really think happiness is crucial to good health and that purpose is a key driver of happiness. But, what if you are still on the path to finding your purpose and want to infuse some happiness into your life right now?

Dr. Becky Su has some words of wisdom: "Happiness is contagious. If for one night only you can be a beacon of happiness and joy, by the end of the night, everyone in your presence will be happy." This is a great reminder that we can find moments of happiness, even during unhappy times, and, just like with love, there's no limit to the amount of happiness there can be in the world.

Dr. Su, whom you've met throughout this book, is perhaps at her most inspiring and helpful when she talks about happiness. Her three steps for happiness are simple and profound:

1. "If you can't change it, don't think about it. If your adult child is struggling and it's something you can't change, don't lose sleep over it. Keep yourself healthy so you can be there for everyone else."

2. "You have to give yourself permission to be happy. You can't make yourself happy, but you can give yourself permission to decide to be happy."

3. "Focus on the beautiful and the good. Your brain is trainable. You're not fixed in your mood, your thinking, or how you feel today or how you'll feel tomorrow. We're wired to notice what's wrong—it's a survival mechanism—but we can counterbalance that instinct. The Chinese philosophers ask the ques-

tion, "Can the monk move the mountain?" The answer is, "What angle do you want to see?"

Being happy is obviously a worthy goal to improve the quality of our lives. But the whole field of happiness research is proving that being happy isn't a "bonus" for a good life; happiness may help us live longer, encourage healthier habits, and even affect our genes. Happiness, in this context, doesn't mean being constantly cheerful or pollyannaish. The goal isn't perfection and doing everything right to be perfectly happy all the time. Happiness coexists with moments of sadness or grief. A rigid adherence to the "right" behaviors— including the habits in this book—doesn't guarantee longevity, and correctness without joy leaves us with a life half lived. Happiness is a way of seeing and interacting with the world that brings positivity, a sense of purpose, and a spark of aliveness that is infectious.

> "MANY TIMES I'VE BEEN TEMPTED. ONE TIME IN THE BIRMINGHAM TRAIN STATION I ACTUALLY BOUGHT A BURGER AND RAISED IT TO MY SALIVATING MOUTH, BUT NEVER TOOK A BITE."
>
> —— Roy Hobbs,
> a 103-year-old vegetarian who regrets
> not eating meat once in awhile

Gratitude Lists

From Oprah Winfrey to Dr. Oz, the powers of gratitude lists are widely hailed. If you never tried, I highly recommend you do. There's no right or wrong way to do it, but many studies have shown that taking time every day to acknowledge the things that make you grateful increases optimism, lowers stress, and increases feelings of joy and contentment. A simple approach is to keep a small notebook next to your bed, write the date, and jot a few notes about what was good and positive in your day—the greeting the barista gave you in the morning, the beautiful sky, the fact that there was a downpour but you didn't ruin your laptop, the e-mail you received from a happy client. Small or large, finding just a few things you're grateful for can shift your mood and perspective.

The Health Effects of Happiness and Positive Attitudes

Research is proving what we've known from experience and observation about the value of purpose, a positive outlook, and finding reasons to be happy even when faced with challenges. For example:

- People who perceive aging as a positive experience are more likely to practice healthy behaviors.

- People who think they're in poor health may die sooner than those who consider themselves healthy (regardless of their actual health status).

- Optimism, hope, life satisfaction, and happiness are associated with lowered likelihood of heart disease and stroke.

Eric Dishman—the cutting-edge researcher who earlier in the book identified the three pillars for medical care, and was largely inspired by his personal experiences taking charge of his life-threatening illness—insisted that happiness be part of his doctors' prescription for his care. He wanted his care to take into account his quality of life, not the quantity. For Dishman, as he explains in his TED talk, that meant a medical plan that goes as follows: *Patient goal: low doses of drugs over longer periods of time, side effects friendly to skiing.*

Dishman believes that his personal "time in snow" therapy has been as important as his drug therapies for his statistics-denying longevity.

Hedonic and Eudaimonic Happiness

If we want to develop our happiness, we need to understand a little more about the aspects of happiness that are most meaningful. Ancient philosophers and modern psychologists talk about *hedonic* and *eudaimonic* happiness. Without doing justice to this rich body of work, the primary distinction between the two forms of happiness is this: hedonic happiness refers to happiness in the moment that is dependent on personal pleasure and satisfaction. Eudaimonic happiness, refers to meaningful experiences that provide engagement, a deep sense of purpose, and lasting fulfillment.

People rated with high levels of eudaimonic happiness showed higher levels of expression of the genes for strong immunity and low inflammation. On the other hand, people rated with high levels of hedonic well-being showed lower levels of expression for genes associated with inflammation and antibody and antiviral protection.

This tells us that as far as health is concerned, we should try to focus less on momentary, hedonic happiness, which may not last very long if the situation changes or the person is facing challenges that make it hard to feel confident, enthusiastic, or lighthearted. Rather, we should seek eudaimonic happiness, which comes from meaning and contributing to the world in some way.

I'm on board with this idea and I hope you'll join me in creating meaningful, lasting happiness in our own lives and in our country.

Connect With Your Inner Child's Purpose to Lift Your Mood

Our attitudes count for a lot when it comes to healthy longevity. It's been shown that if you believe you look and feel younger than your actual biological age, you're likely to live longer than someone who feels his or her age or even older. Becca Levy, PhD, a researcher on aging at Yale School of Public Health, has shown that a positive attitude toward aging can help you live, on average, 7.5 years longer. Our beliefs about aging—whether we think of it in terms of limitation and inevitable decline or in terms of lifelong potential and living at the edge of our capacity—shape our actual health.

At our Aegis Living communities, we've discovered that people who live longer and happier lives seem to have some kind of totem that connects them to their younger selves. One resident who was nearly 90 loved to ride the Ferris wheel every year. Another resident, who held many weight lifting records, continued to lift weights at 91 years old. Many residents remind me of my mother, who believed dancing was her fountain of youth and that dressing young helped keep her young. At Aegis Headquarters I built a tree house behind the main building so my staff has easy access to childlike experiences now and again.

But the opposite seems true as well. People who think they are "too old" for certain activities they might enjoy and need to "look and act their age" seem to age prematurely.

Your Longevity Is in Your Hands

If you equate aging with inactivity or being "over the hill," you're less likely to take care of yourself. You'll give in to decline. If you believe that aging is defined by how you feel, you're more likely to practice the habits of health, creating a healthier life span. You'll eat foods that fuel rather than harm your body. You'll get the restorative sleep you need so you have the vitality to fuel yourself throughout the day. You'll move more and sit less.

All these habits will help you feel better—and younger—and, in turn, help you have the best possible health for the rest of your life.

Your Healthy Edge

DEVELOPING YOUR PURPOSE

Having a strong purpose in your life leads to better moods and increased happiness, especially as we age. The suggestions below can help you further nurture your life's purpose to increase your happiness and chances for living a long and healthy life.

- [ ] Make happiness contagious when you're around others (e.g., smile at them, compliment them, offer them help should they need it).

- [ ] Give yourself permission to be happy even if those around you are not.

- [ ] Consider doing activities that gave you purpose as a child (e.g., riding Ferris wheels or horses, being on a boat, or roller skating).

- [ ] Make a mood board to reflect your life's purpose.

- [ ] Journal to determine what your life's purpose is (e.g., helping raise your grandkids, furthering an environmental cause, running a 10-minute mile when you are 80, or making people laugh).

- [ ] Boost your moods by getting quality sleep, walking outside, doing yoga, or meditating.

Notes

I imagine that everyone reading this book has been on his or her life's journey for quite some time. Not one of us knows how long we will live and what will happen tomorrow. We may be at the halfway mark, the three-quarters mark, or in our final days.

But if I've learned anything on my journey through life—including the writing of this book—it's that we shape our future and health every day. Our joy and purpose, our friends, our intellectual pursuits, and our care for our bodies and well-being all have a profound impact on how well and how long we live.

As someone who started out as a traditional meat-and-potatoes guy trying to become a success and found myself in my 50s reinventing the way I lived, I know the journey has many twist and turns. I subjected my brain to electric impulse treatments (to improve memory and recall). I tried testosterone injections for longevity (not for me). I've had my genome mapped, measured, dissected, and reconstructed. I've had regular blood work to refine my personalized vitamin and supplement program, and I've charted my vitals and my steps and my REM sleep.

Net-net, I'm now 50 pounds lighter and have the sense that I'm 50 times more alive. I've held on to the best approaches for me and let go of the rest—and I keep learning.

With lots of supportive health professionals, family, and friends, and a steady embrace of the habits of health, I've freed myself from an unsustainable regimen of antacids, inhalers, steroids, and blood pressure pills. I can honestly say I'm not miserable about my health or worried about the future. I have a new view of the decades to come. Happiness is becoming a habit, just like work has been my whole life.

Robin Williams, that master of creativity and passion, knew that joy, laughter, and passion were gifts he could share with the world. They were at the center of his career and life as he struggled with a devastating illness that was only diagnosed after his death. In the 1996 movie *Jack,* Williams plays the character of a boy in a man's body due to a rare condition. At age 10 he looks like a 40-year-old, and he confronts all the challenges of being different. At the end of the movie, and as the end of Jack's life nears, he gives a valedictorian speech to be remembered for all time. He tells his classmates not to worry so much because life is fleeting. He asks them, if they ever get distressed, to look up at the velvety black sky and make a wish on a star. Finally, he leaves his friends with this goal, "Make your life spectacular. I know I did. I made it, Mom. I'm a grown-up."

That's my parting wish for you. I want you to put *spectacular* on your bucket list, whatever that is. Yes, say goodbye to sugar. Yes, make movement and mindfulness your mantras. Yes, begin eating in a new way, or try your first cleanse. And yes, keep making new friends.

> MAKE YOUR LIFE BE SPECTACULAR. I KNOW I DID. I MADE IT, MOM. I'M A GROWN-UP.

But don't get overwhelmed by all the "shoulds." Don't get overwhelmed or paralyzed with all the information out there on how to be healthy. Don't be hard on yourself if your habits flag and you need to start again. Your health starts with simple steps, and each small step can make a big difference. So don't worry. Just do something today to improve your odds of experiencing more health for more years.

Be guided by your purpose and by joy—and what makes life spectacular to you. Let yourself let go of missed opportunities, regrets, and the pains of life. Get out in the sun, enjoy life, take a walk, call a friend. This is the path that will lead you to the best, healthiest life possible.

Remember that you have the power, more now than ever, to take charge of your health and longevity. You are the driver, and the ownership manual is in your hands, literally.

Make your life spectacular,
Dwayne

Microhabits

BITE-SIZED ACTIONS MAKE ALL THE DIFFERENCE

I've found it's the little things I do that help me stay engaged with my health and don't make it all feel overwhelming. The microhabits I practice are listed below, and I recommend you pick five to 10 and see if you can stick to them for 30 days.

TAKING CHARGE

1. I became, and still am, a voracious consumer of medical information. This helps me better understand my body and how I can help it stay healthy.

2. My mornings are totally different now. I have a full routine that I follow each morning to help me have the best day possible. It's all listed in the next section called "Starting Your Day Right."

3. Every week I get massage and acupuncture to keep my body's healing powers strong.

CLEARING THE SYSTEM

4. I purposefully eliminate toxic buildup in my body so it doesn't cloud my brain. I do this through hydration, the right foods, fiber … anything so my body doesn't get stuck.

5. Four times a year I do a 21-day cleanse to rid my body of toxins and let it heal.

6. I practice transcendental meditation twice each day to cleanse my brain, increase my energy, and reduce overall stress in my body.

7. I have a place I like to go to get away and consciously unplug from technology and all the noise in my life.

8. To improve cellular protection and remove toxins from my body, I take four to five cleansing breaths a day.

EATING, HYDRATION, AND NUTRITION

9. I didn't think food could make me sick. To get better, I had to become a conscious eater.

10. Subconscious eating and having access to any food in any amount was a big problem for me. One habit I developed in retraining myself to eat is to take one bite of food, wait for two minutes, and then ask myself, "How hungry am I really?"

11. Measuring on a scale of 1 to 10 (with 10 being full), I stop eating at a 5.5 and nibble off my plate after that.

12. Reducing sugar and dairy helped immensely. When I'd eat those two things together, it set off an inflammation storm in my body. I *love* ice cream, so eliminating dairy and most sugar was a big microhabit for me to develop. Now I eat a small bowl of good-quality ice cream once in a while.

13. I try to go to bed a little bit hungry each night so I know my body has more opportunity to rest and release toxins.

14. When you eat, you're performing a chemistry experiment. I carefully choose which foods I want to eat in the same meal. It took a lot of experimentation and discipline to do that.

15. Ketchup was an everyday thing in my diet. I had to give it up because of its sugar and acid.

16. I was a "pure white" eater. Now I eat much more color. All the vitamins are in the color.

17. To encourage cell replenishment, I make superfoods part of my daily diet. These include eggs, spinach, broccoli, avocados, and green tea.

18. I take a close look at foods that have been labeled as bad, things like salt and butter. There are butters (European) and salts (Hawaiian) that are better for you.

19. To clear brain fog, clear dizziness, and even lower my blood pressure, I drink eight ounces of water every morning first thing. It works. The body really needs this lubrication to work well. I try to drink 70 to 80 ounces of water a day to pee gin clear.

20. Off the drugstore shelf was the way I used to buy my vitamins. Now I'm on the personalized vitamin kick and it's not much more expensive than the ones off the shelf.

21. Gut health is essential to longevity, so I take a good-quality probiotic every day.

22. There's a supplement called NAD (nicotinamide adenine dinucleotide) I take to reverse mitochondrial decay. It improves the molecular structure of cells and gives me more energy.

23. Steak was my friend. Now I limit eating red meat to once or twice a month.

24. The right kind of fish is a mainstay in my diet now. I eat it in moderation to avoid any buildup of mercury and other toxins.

25. Men love their cereal, and I loved a mixing bowl full of it with peanut butter on top. I had to say goodbye to it, but I'm much better off without it.

MOVEMENT

26. These days I lift weights that are less heavy but with more reps. This is better for tone and range of motion.

27. Tai chi is something I practice for balance. I also stand on one foot when brushing my teeth.

28. To protect my joints, I stopped trying to run miles and miles. Now I run three- to four-minute intervals and then walk. I also use an elliptical machine, plus I bike, swim, walk, and hike.

SLEEP

29. I really analyze my sleep. If my REM is less than 1.5 hours and my deep sleep is less than 1.15 hours, I suffer—my thinking, my energy, my balance, everything.

30. Napping is important. I nap 10 to 15 minutes three to four times a week, especially if I have an event at night.

31. Relationships, purpose, emotions, and good relationships equal happiness. Beyond sleep, relationships are the second most important thing, in my opinion, to increase health and longevity.

32. Toxic energy and toxic people destroy cells, so I intentionally got out of toxic relationships.

33. To increase my happiness, I try to stay in the moment and adore the things I have instead of longing for things I want. That's hard because I'm a futurist.

34. Children and younger people can have amazing medicinal effects, so I seek relationships with younger people and children.

35. The small stuff doesn't get me upset anymore, and I try not to get stressed out over things that aren't crucial.

36. I give myself permission to cry to release emotional tension and help lower my blood pressure.

Starting Your Day Right

Before you get out of bed:

- Wiggle each finger and toe, and then rotate your ankles while you are lying down in bed to get your blood moving.

- Slowly sit up.

- Sit in bed for two to three minutes and take three deep breaths, exhaling slowly for each breath.

- Drink the water you put by your bed the night before.

Before breakfast:

- Go to the bathroom, and don't turn on your TV or reach for your phone or tablet when you are done.

- Give thanks for the morning. Look outside and consciously focus on one element of nature—a tree, a plant, or a flower—and give thanks to the Earth.

- Take deep breaths and reach up and do a full-body stretch.

- After being awake for at least 30 minutes, meditate for 15 to 20 minutes.

- Eat breakfast. You can eat before meditation if you need to.

Before taking a shower:

- Take a walk outside and focus on three things for which you are grateful. It could be for feeling healthy, a fulfilling relationship, or the fresh air.

- Be conscious of the nature you see as you walk.

- If nature can't be part of your walk, try focusing on something that pleases you—your manicure, your comfortable shoes, or the people around you. This helps you be present.

Before you charge into your day:

- When you return from your walk, shower and let the warm water run on places of your body that need healing. Feel the pulsating water pleasing, warming, and healing your body.

- Towel off and say three times, "This will be a wonderful day!"

- Lay out clothes that fit you well and make you feel marvelous, and then get dressed.

- After getting dressed, think of a color that you love. Imagine that color engulfing you, and see this color as a protective layer that shields you from any negativity out in the world.

Now, go start your day.

Dwayne's Healthy Habits in Order of Importance

Over the years, I've learned that there are layers of action that lead to health and longevity. My hierarchy may be different than yours, but I thought it might save you some time, or give you a place to start, if you see how I prioritize the wellness efforts in my life.

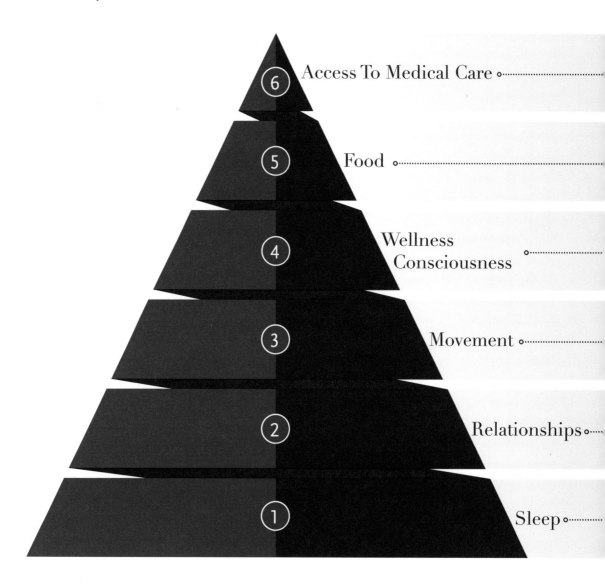

6 Access To Medical Care

5 Food

4 Wellness Consciousness

3 Movement

2 Relationships

1 Sleep

I GET MY REGULAR CHECKUPS AND HEALTH SCREENINGS.
I ALSO VISIT PRACTITIONERS THAT TREAT MY WHOLE BODY.

EATING IS A CHEMISTRY EXPERIMENT IN THE BODY.
I KNOW WHICH FOODS HURT AND HELP MINE.

BECAUSE I DOCUMENT MY HEALTH STATUS DAILY,
I AM AN EXPERT ON MY OWN HEALTH.

MOVING IS CRUCIAL TO KEEPING ME
MOVING AS AS I AGE.

I DEVELOP RELATIONSHIPS WITH PEOPLE I LIKE.
I END TOXIC RELATIONSHIPS.

THE FOUNDATION OF MY HEALTH
IS GETTING A GOOD NIGHTS SLEEP.

1. Sleep

Quality sleep is extremely important for good health and longevity. It's when the brain and body cleanse themselves of toxins and create new, healthy cells.

Invest in your bedding and bedroom so that both make you feel comfortable and at peace.

Unplug two hours before you go to sleep.

Get a sleep tracker and log your deep and REM sleep. Initially see if you can get one hour of deep sleep each night.

2. Relationships, Purpose, and Happiness

Close relationships create happiness that in turn feeds the body and brain. People who know they are needed—those who have a purpose—tend to live healthier, longer lives.

Take the time to do enjoyable activities with your good friends. Don't put it off.

Consider calling a friend instead of texting.

Find a way to create a friendship with one person 20 years younger than you.

Extract yourself from toxic relationships, including at work, at home, and with friends.

If you don't have a bucket list, make one and commit to checking it off bit by bit over the years.

Take action on deep desires to give you wonderful reasons to be needed and to get out of bed each morning, especially after you retire.

3. Movement

Think about moving rather than exercising. The modern gym is an American concept. The rest of the world moves to stay fit.

Get a device that tracks your steps. Learn what your average steps per day are and what you can do to double that number.

Commit to getting more movement around your home (gardening, cooking, walking the dog, not sitting down until 8 pm to watch TV).

Find ways to move at work (walking meetings, taking the stairs, using restrooms on a different floor).

4. Wellness Consciousness

Be an expert on your health. Knowing your body better than your doctor lets you take charge of your health and health care.

Purchase a scale, blood pressure cuff, and glucometer (if you are concerned about diabetes).

Test and record each number—weight, blood pressure, and blood sugar—every morning to learn your trends. Document your movement and food for the day and indicate how they impact you.

Bring all your data to doctor appointments and prepare for the appointments like you would for and run a business meeting. This helps doctors with limited time get to an accurate diagnosis faster.

5. Food

Food can hurt you, so it's important to understand which foods are helping and hurting your body. Obvious and hidden sugars in the diet are the biggest culprits. Other foods, and food combinations, can negatively impact your health as well.

Write down the foods you know upset your body. Avoid those, and sugar, for 30 days. Document the results (weight loss, better sleep, less gas/nausea/bloating).

Time how long it takes you to eat dinner. Over the course of a month, see if you can add one minute a night to your eating time.

Make an appointment with a nutritionist to get your blood work tested for nutritional imbalances and to learn which foods are best and worst for you.

Consider taking personalized vitamins.

6. Access to Medical Care

Take advantage of the preventive visits and screenings your medical benefits offer. Also work with highly respected medical practitioners trained to treat the body as a whole and improve your body's own healing powers (acupuncture, integrative-functional medicine, nutrition, massage). Before you make an appointment, do your research on the medical practitioner you want to see. Look into his or her background, reputation, and any past or pending litigation.

Call and schedule a meet-and-greet appointment to "try before you buy."

The day before your appointment, make a list of questions and requests for your doctor.

Index